40 plus

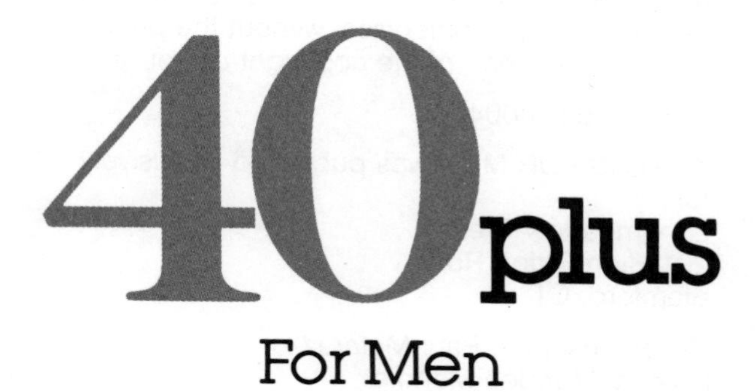

For Men

Your Guide to a Healthy Body and Mind

By Richard Amdur

LONGMEADOW PRESS

ISBN: 0-681-40048-X

40 PLUS FOR MEN was published exclusively for
Longmeadow Press
201 High Ridge Road
Stamford, CT

Cover Designer: Paul Matarazzo
Design: Meridee Mandio

Typeset by Paragraphics

Cover color separation by South Seas Graphic Art Co.

Printed and bound in Hong Kong by Leefung-Asco Printers Ltd.

Digit on the right indicates the number of this printing.
10 9 8 7 6 5 4 3 2 1

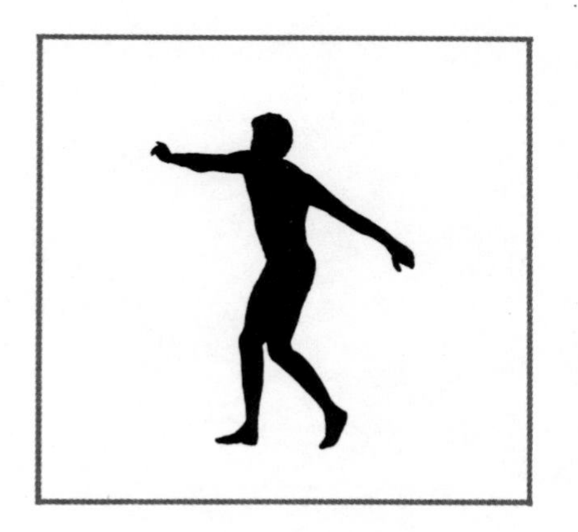

CONTENTS

Introduction

Life Begins at 40

We are living in a new age. "Health food," once an alternative associated primarily with the counterculture, has become decidedly mainstream—nowadays even fast-food restaurants sport salad bars. Meanwhile, exercise enthusiasts jam health clubs and city parks morning, noon, and night, pushing themselves to new heights of fitness. An era of unprecedented physical awareness is upon us, and it makes perfectly good sense.

The health boom has perhaps made its biggest impact on middle-aged Americans, those men and women between the ages of 40 and 65 who have decided to take control of aging before it takes control of them. They know that staying young has more to do with how they take care of their bodies and how they feel about themselves than with their actual chronological age. And by educating themselves about what's good for their bodies and then getting out and doing those good things, the over-40s are living their peak years at their best. Instead of bemoaning their "fate," the men and women over 40 are turning mid-life into the prime of life.

Chances are you don't feel as fit as you did in your 20s, but there is no reason you couldn't. It is never too late to take control, never too late to make both your body and your mind fulfill their potential. Men over 40 are society's pacesetters—the leaders of business, politics, and industry, husbands and fathers, men of wisdom and maturity. Your physical self can express all that and more.

Never before has so much attention been paid to the health and fitness needs of mature adults. Never before have there been so many compelling reasons for a man to approach his post-40 years with such enthusiasm and optimism. Many of the over-40 set have already woken up to this fact; for them life has never been better. The goal of *40 PLUS for Men* is to spread the word even further, to show *you* how to be over 40 and proud of it.

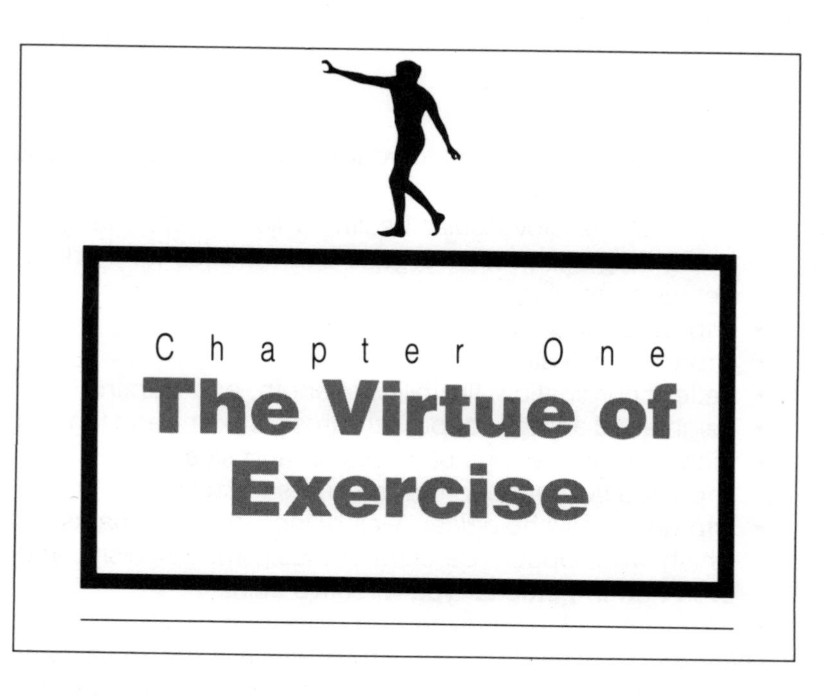

Chapter One
The Virtue of Exercise

The nationwide fitness boom is not just a fad, nor is it solely a young person's pursuit. Men and women over 40 are amply represented among the legions of runners, swimmers, bicyclists, and others who are convinced—for excellent reasons—that regular exercise is crucial to one's overall well-being. One could even say that men and women over 40 are the phenomenon's leading spokespersons: Jane Fonda, George Burns, and many others have all written best-selling fitness, health, and beauty guides. And millions of men over 40 have discovered that exercise means leading longer, happier lives. Shouldn't you be among them?

Exercise, in tandem with proper dietary habits (see Chapter Two), is a remarkably direct way to enhance your prospects for sound health and mental well-being well into your later years. When exercise is performed on a regular basis, the benefits you are likely to derive include:

- weight loss or maintenance of your ideal weight (Developing proper nutritional habits is an essential complement to exercise and important to your health whether or not you are very active.)

- improved cardiovascular health, which means that your heart, lungs, and other organs and muscles will work together more efficiently
- improved musculoskeletal health
- improved digestion
- better coordination, flexibility, strength, and stamina
- heightened ability to cope with stress, anxiety, and tension
- more fulfilling periods of relaxation and sleep
- improved sexual performance and satisfaction
- improved psychological well-being, the hallmarks of which will probably be extra enthusiasm, optimism, and even new impetus for your creative spirit
- an easier end to smoking and other bad habits

There is no real mystery as to why exercise is such a salutary pursuit. The body can be likened to an automobile or any other sophisticated machine that must be kept finely tuned in order to perform at its best. If you want your senses to remain keen, if you want to be strong, durable, graceful—in short, if you want to be a physically capable human being for your *entire* life, as we are designed to be—you must keep your body well conditioned through physical activity. It's that simple.

The Aging Process

Aging induces some potentially dismaying physiological changes in a man's body, but they need not frighten you once you understand them. Generally, the older you get the harder it is for your brain, central nervous system, cardiovascular system, and musculoskeletal system to maintain their optimum working order (which means that you just have to pay more attention to the way you treat your body).

Doctors agree that at some time around the age of 30 signs of the body's decline begin to become increasingly evident. The amount of blood pumped by the heart begins to decrease.

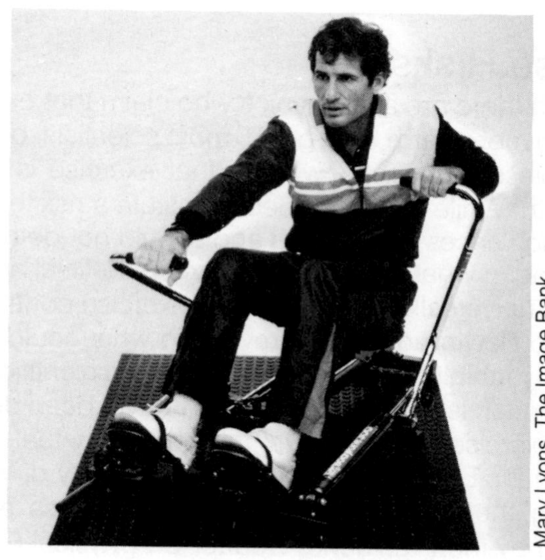

Marv Lyons, The Image Bank

The number and size of muscle fibers and nerve cells decline, lessening the body's strength and speed. Agility suffers, as do endurance and respiration—what doctors call "vital capacity." Excess fat seems to accumulate more easily—usually around the midriff. In fact, the changes are more extensive than this brief list indicates. At one stage or another, aging and its associated processes take their toll on virtually every aspect of one's functioning. Overall, according to C.P. Gilmore, author of *Exercise for Fitness,* "the body's capacity to do work (defined as any task requiring physical exertion) declines by the age of 75 to less than half its capacity at age 20."

But it is important to note that aging is not the sole "cause" of decreased bodily functioning. Among the other significant factors involved in your body's aging process are lifestyle habits (e.g., if you are a sedentary person) and the incidence of disease. The goal of *40 Plus* is to help you focus on those factors—namely lifestyle (which includes preventive health care)—that you can control.

Exercise Risks?

Although there are a few cynics who claim that exercise can actually do more harm than good, most scientists, doctors and health professionals acknowledge that exercise is the key to good health. While exercise does constitute a risk to some individuals such cases are isolated and should not deter one from participating in what is predominantly a beneficial activity.

There is universally little doubt that exercise contributes significantly to slowing down or preventing what could otherwise be seriously inhibiting bodily changes. The scientific evidence saying as much is in your favor. (It has not yet been determined if regular exercise has the power to affect the actual aging process itself.) Dr. Everet L. Smith of the University of Wisconsin, addressing the National Conference on Fitness and Aging sponsored by the President's Council on Physical Fitness and Sports in 1981, said, "Individuals who maintain a high degree of physical activity have a functional capacity 20 to 30 percent greater than that of the average individual their age. Physical capacity declines at a very rapid rate, however, with cessation of chronic physical activity."

In another, more dramatic, study discussed at the same conference by Dr. Herbert A. DeVries of the University of Southern California, functional losses similar to those seen in a 75-year-old man were induced in young, well-conditioned men simply by forcing them to endure three weeks of bed rest. As DeVries commented: "Thus we might say that changes roughly equal to thirty years of aging have been brought about by simply putting the organism at rest and not allowing any physical exercise."

Many men, faced with the jarring physical manifestation of aging, surrender to the "over-the-hill" myth. Not you! As the evidence attests, it is completely within your power to alter your lifestyle (or to build upon your present habits) so as to set the stage for an exciting and vigorous life ahead. For most men, the most important place to start is with the heart.

Cardiovascular Fitness

Foremost among the special health and fitness needs of men over 40 is keeping their heart and cardiovascular system in good shape, because heart and blood vessels wear with age, making the body more susceptible to heart attack, stroke, congestive heart failure, and high blood pressure.

Consider these statistics: According to the American Heart Association, nearly one million Americans died from heart or blood-vessel disease in 1983, almost as many as from all other causes of death combined. Over sixty-three million people—more than one out of every four Americans—suffer some form of heart disease. Figures from the Framingham Heart Study—a long-running, comprehensive study of that Massachusetts town's population—are equally stark. They show that a man in his early 40s has one chance in eight of developing heart disease within fourteen years, a man in his late 40s has one chance in six, and a man in his early 50s has one chance in five. As Dr. William Castelli, director of the study, told *Science Digest,* "These are not old fogies dying of coronary disease. These are young fogies, men in their 40s and 50s. This is the American epidemic." He is right—heart disease has been the country's leading cause of death since 1910.

These findings are dismaying, to be sure, but they do not need to be frightening. They need not condemn you to a life of fear. Recent research (including the Framingham study) has shown that **heart problems are not an inevitable consequence of age but rather are more likely the result of the way people live.** Furthermore, a study conducted by the National Institute of Aging shows that, contrary to popular belief, the actual physical functioning of the heart does not necessarily decline as a person ages. Previously it was thought that heart function declined 1 percent per year after age 20. What these results suggest is that it is easily within your power to keep your heart working well.

Proof of this can be found in another statistic—this one much more encouraging: **The death rate from heart attack has dropped a remarkable 37 percent in the last twenty years.** In the 1980s, according to *50 Plus* magazine, "the lives of 300,000 men and women are being saved each year." Among the reasons most often cited for this dramatic success in the fight against heart disease are improved dietary awareness, more effective stress management, and the fitness boom—all instances in which individuals asserted control over their destinies.

To many people, runner/author Jim Fixx was—until he died—the epitome of the exercise phenomenon. Once an overweight, inactive smoker, Fixx took up jogging with something of a vengeance and turned himself into a championship-class long-distance runner. His best-selling *The Complete Book of Running*—in which he documented his physical transformation and offered a thorough guide to the sport—was instrumental in popularizing jogging and the exercise phenomenon in general.

It was only after he suffered a fatal heart attack, at the age of 52, while jogging (throwing joggers and exercise enthusiasts into a panic), that his congenital heart ailment was made public. Fixx's father had died of heart failure at the age of 43, and Fixx himself had such severe arterial blockage that doctors said not only that he should have had a bypass operation but also that he might have died whether or not he had been jogging.

Nonetheless, doctors estimated that his extensive training had granted him an extra nine years of life, and he remains an inspiring figure. His only apparent mistake was ignoring the advice of friends who had implored him to see a physician. (It's a mistake no man over 40 can afford to make.)

Less than a month after Fixx's death, doctors at Stanford and Harvard universities unveiled the first scientific evidence that exercise **prolongs** life (earlier links between exercise and longevity had been considered lacking in scientific underpinning). **Among the study's findings was that men who regularly exercised had about half as many heart attacks as those who did**

not. As Dr. Bruce B. Dan told *The New York Times,* "The real discovery of this research is not that people who exercise have strong cardiovascular systems; rather it is that sedentary people have shriveled hearts and most of us who do not exercise have an atrophied body."

Although exercise cannot completely eliminate heart trouble, it does significantly lessen the likelihood of your falling prey to the disease. It does this by strengthening the heart and acting against some of the leading risk factors for heart disease: high blood-cholesterol levels, high blood pressure, obesity, and stress.

Strengthen Your Heart

Since the heart is a muscle, it is made stronger by the rhythmic muscular activity characteristic of exercise (especially aerobic exercise), which increases blood flow through the heart and heightens demand on the heart's muscle fibers. For the heart, stronger means being able to pump more oxygenated blood to the body with each beat; a strengthened heart doesn't have to work as hard to do this, and thus will probably last longer. In addition, there are indications that exercise actually fosters the growth of new networks of small blood vessels in the heart, enhancing the heart's ability to transport oxygen efficiently.

Exercise and Cholesterol

But exercise is beneficial to your heart in other ways as well. Many researchers, physicians, and nutritionists have said that cholesterol may be the number-one risk factor in heart disease. And as a man ages his arteries are more likely to become clogged with fatty deposits—such as cholesterol—which can then restrict or even halt the flow of blood, ultimately causing a heart attack or stroke. According to the American Heart Association, over 50 percent of middle-aged men have levels of cholesterol in their blood that place them close to the "high risk" category for coronary heart disease. Controlling your diet (see Chapter Two) can reduce the amount of cholesterol buildup;

Activity	Calories Consumed Per ½ Hour
Bicycling, 15 mph	360
Running, 6 mph	350
Swimming, freestyle	260
Jumping rope	250
Tennis (singles)	220
Walking, 4 mph	160
Tennis (doubles)	160
Golf (walking)	150

Based on a Weight Level of 150 Pounds

Decrease or Increase by 10% for Every 15 Pounds Difference in Weight.

but exercise can increase the ratio of "good" cholesterol (that cholesterol which is needed by the body to build cell walls and for other functions) to "bad" cholesterol in the blood, thus having a mitigating effect on an undesirable buildup.

Lowering Blood Pressure

High blood pressure, also known as hypertension and called "a silent killer" by many because it has no specific symptoms and no early-warning signs, commonly afflicts men over 40 and can lead to more serious health hazards. It weakens the heart's pumping efficiency as well as the heart and arteries in general.

A normal blood-pressure reading for an adult male might be 120/80—the first number being the systolic pressure (the pressure of the blood flow when the heart beats), and the second number being the diastolic pressure (the pressure of the blood's flow between heartbeats). The American Heart Association defines high blood pressure as a "systolic pressure greater than or equal to 140 and/or a diastolic pressure greater than or equal to 90." The measurements are taken by a sphygmomanometer, the rubber-cuffed instrument with which almost everyone is familiar. You should have your blood pressure checked at least once a year after age 40.

Exercising to maintain a strong heart is one way of controlling blood pressure. And yoga practitioners claim that deep-breathing techniques and rhythmical motions have a naturally tranquilizing effect on an individual, thus lowering blood pressure. However, medication and dietary alterations, such as decreasing one's intake of cholesterol, salt, and alcohol are the primary treatment for high blood pressure.

Obesity and Stress

The ill effects of obesity and stress are obviously lessened through constant exercise—the former through weight loss and the latter through the release of tension that accompanies most exercise. Obesity's role in heart disease has been demonstrably established: **One study showed that men who weighed 20 percent or more than their ideal weight were three times as likely to suffer heart attacks**—findings that are generally attributed to the fact that excess weight places an additional strain on the heart. Stress, meanwhile, is linked to heart conditions, particularly high blood pressure because of its general ability to disrupt the body's functioning. Cardiac specialists all emphasize the importance of adequate stress management. (See pages 111–117 for more information on stress.)

Aerobics—Exercise for the Heart

Exercise is obviously the cornerstone of cardiovascular fitness. But what type of exercise is best? Health professionals, including the American Heart Association, agree that aerobic training should be the basis of all fitness programs. Among the sports considered aerobic are: swimming, hiking, bicycling, cross-country skiing, rope jumping, vigorous walking, jogging, rowing, and bench stepping. And at least one exercise expert has called swimming "the closest thing yet to the anti-aging pill."

Dr. Kenneth Cooper, who is not only credited with starting the worldwide jogging phenomenon but also with introducing aerobics to America, says that the top five aerobic exercises, in order, are: cross-country skiing, swimming, running, cycling, and walking. The factors that these activities have in common is that all involve prolonged, repetitive, and demanding physical exertion that forces the body to improve its ability to transport oxygen.

Sports such as weight lifting, tennis, baseball, and touch football, which consist largely of stops and starts, are not aerobic, even though they are athletic. Indeed, as one doctor says, "If the only exercise you do is play tennis . . . in which you go from a dead stop to full exertion in three or four steps, you may put a serious strain on your heart."

Your aerobic-exercise program should be consistently performed at least three times a week for several months if any benefits are to be derived. Adding calisthenics and weight training to supplement your aerobic regimen is, of course, a terrific way to achieve a fit body, but be aware that neither of these activities alone is beneficial enough to constitute an entire program. In other words, they will not strengthen your heart.

Warm-up and cool-down periods of about ten minutes' duration should bracket your workout. Without warm-ups or cool-downs you are in danger of harming your body—not helping it. Cool-downs are particularly important for cardiovascular health. If you stop exercising abruptly your blood pressure drops too quickly, causing the amount of the hormones epinephrine and norepinephrine in your blood to rise dramatically. This can cause *arrhythmia,* an irregular heartbeat.

Home equipment such as stationary "exer-cycles" and rowing machines are perfectly fine for an at-home workout since they give you an aerobic workout. But be sure that these machines comfortably accommodate your frame; otherwise, you

Monitoring Your Heart Rate

Your target heart rate varies according to your age. The best time to check is immediately after a steady aerobic workout of at least 20 to 30 minutes. To monitor your heart rate, take your pulse by placing one finger over the carotid artery in your neck or the radial artery in your wrist. Count your pulse for 6 seconds and multiply by 10. You know you're achieving proper aerobic benefits (and thus becoming more fit) from the exercise if your pulse is close to the target rate for your age.

Age	Maximum Heart Rate	Target Heart Rate
35	185	130
40	180	126
45	175	123
50	170	119
55	165	116
60	160	112
65	155	109
70	150	105
80	145	98

could damage your back. If you don't have room to work out at home or simply prefer going to a health club of some sort, one alternative that is particularly appropriate for heart health is a cardio-fitness center. These offer individualized, completely supervised exercise programs—using treadmills, bicycles, rowing machines, Universal equipment, and more—that are geared toward improving cardiovascular fitness and health in general. Programs are monitored on a daily basis and are adjusted based on your progress. Basic nutritional guidance is also offered.

Cardio-fitness centers are staffed with trained experts in various related fields. Furthermore, the close attention these experts give to each member makes such fitness centers better than most health clubs, where a member is, more or less, on his own. As might be expected, however, cardio-fitness centers are more expensive than health clubs. But if you or your doctor feels you need a very disciplined program—either preventive or rehabilitative—enrolling in one might be worth considering. *Note:* Cardio-fitness centers cater to men of all ages, whether or not they are in shape.

Heart Tests

Keep in mind that for some people working out can be a health risk. You should always consult your physician before undertaking anything strenuous, especially if you've been inactive for a long period of time or have had any serious ailments.

Even if you're healthy you may simply be curious (and wisely cautious) about how your heart, blood vessels, and circulatory system are faring. There are many heart tests that are available. (see Chapter Two for more details), If you have any known medical problems, family history of heart disease, or have not exercised in a while, some of these tests are an absolute must. Since they differ in cost and effectiveness, a doctor's advice should be sought as to which is best for you.

For the healthy man over 40, the tests include:

- a heredity check, to see if any members of your family have suffered from heart disease
- a blood-pressure test
- a cholesterol test
- a resting EKG, which monitors the heart's electrical currents in order to detect any abnormalities or damage.
- an exercise stress test, which tests your pulse both at rest and after some form of exercise (usually a step test). This measures your heart's capacity for activity.
- a forced vital capacity test, in which you gauge the strength of your heart and lungs by breathing deeply into a machine called a spirometer, which then measures the total volume of your exhalation.

For the man with already-diagnosed heart abnormalities or other physical problems, the tests include:

- an exercise stress test.
- a thallium scan, in which tracer dye is injected into the body through the arm and read by a scintillation camera to determine the heart's efficiency.
- an angiogram (also known as an arteriogram), which is an X ray of the heart in action taken after a dye is injected into the body (since X rays don't pick up organs) and read through the use of a special tube inserted into the body. This test takes up to 3 hours and requires the use of sedatives, since the person tested must remain still for the duration of the procedure.
- a cardiac catheterization, another way for investigators to see the heart in action through the use of a special tube that is inserted into the body.

Exercise: for the Heart and More

Aside from the importance of maintaining one's ideal weight for reasons of heart health (and as a means of combating other diseases), staying trim and free of excess fat is a goal in and of itself. You will not only look better—to yourself and to others—but chances are when your body has been shaped and formed to its optimum weight and balance you'll also perform better at everything you do.

Men over 40 facing the problem of accumulated excess fat should be aware of several things:

- **Exercise burns excess fat.** While some amount of fat is needed by the body as insulation and padding, excess fat has been implicated not only in heart disease but also in diabetes, gall bladder problems, and gout. Dieting, on the other hand, more often leads to the loss of water and active tissue, both of which are crucial to the normal functioning of bones and joints. And dieting alone usually causes a slowdown of your basal metabolic rate, making losing

Three-Minute Stamina Test

For this test, you'll need a stopwatch and a sturdy platform—eight inches high—to serve as a step. You'll need to step at a constant tempo, so a metronome set at 96 is helpful. However, a friend calling out or clapping the rhythm, or watching the stopwatch, should keep you stepping in time. *Warning:* If while taking the test you experience shortness of breath, dizziness, or any pain, stop immediately. Consult your doctor before trying again or exercising.

1. Step up first with one foot, then with the other. Next, step down with the first foot and then with the second. Repeat the cycle once every 2½ seconds (if you have a metronome, move one foot at every beat). After 3 minutes sit down and rest for 30 seconds without talking.
2. After resting, lightly place three fingertips on your neck, just beneath your jawbone and to one side of your Adam's apple or on the inside of your wrist. Using the stopwatch, count for 30 seconds the number of throbs you feel in the larger artery under your fingertips.
3. Find in the column of figures that applies to your age the number of heartbeats that you counted and discover your fitness level.

Heartbeat Count after Step Test

Fitness Level	Age 40–49	Age 50 and Over
Excellent	40 or less	41 or less
Good	41–44	42–45
Fair	45–52	46–52
Poor	53 or more	53 or more

weight more difficult.

- **Men lose 3 to 5 percent of their active tissue (muscle) each decade after age 25,** which means that unless men also lose 3 to 5 percent of their total weight, excess fat becomes a real problem. And since your basal metabolic rate slows down in middle age, it's easy to put on *fat* while you're losing *muscle.*
- **Most excess fat on men seems to settle around the midriff,** placing stress on several major joints and muscles, including your heart. Upper-body fat is much more harmful to your health than lower-body fat. Exercise not only helps remove the weight creating the stress but also strengthens the muscles in these troubled spots.
- **Exercise relieves fatigue.** It's very simple. Exercise relieves fatigue because the muscles and joints become conditioned to do more work before tiring.
- **Exercise releases stress.** Tension increases the activity of the muscles' sensory receptors, which in turn overloads the nervous system with information in the form of electrical impulses. Exercise decreases the activity of these receptors, inducing a calmed, less-frenetic state.
- **Your emotional well-being greatly benefits from regular exercise.** Most people often feel something of an euphoric or ecstatic feeling after exercising, or at the very least a lessening of any depressive tendencies. Although biological processes (your brain releases *endorphins,* which cause a natural "high") may also be contributing to this sensation, it is clear that the psychological component is equally important. Putting your body into shape is a confidence builder, an occasion in which you can take control of your life, a true achievement that has the positive effect on other areas of life—most notably work, interpersonal relationships, and self-awareness. This is particularly important to the over-40 man who is adjusting to new levels of professional achievement, new stages in his marriage or

love life, and other emotional changes associated with this time of life.

Low-Stress Fitness

For all the miracles it can bring about, exercise is not something that any man over 40 should just jump into, especially if he has been inactive. If you've basically led a sedentary lifestyle up until now, forget the "no pain, no gain" adage. A better motto would be "easy does it," and that means low-stress fitness. In low-stress fitness the emphasis is on warming up—with lots of stretching—and cooling down while gradually building up an aerobic workout.

Low-stress fitness fans are high on these aerobics: walking, cycling, and swimming. Walking is the most natural of all the aerobic exercises, and what's more, it can combine exercise with fresh air and sightseeing. Running, on the other hand, can be very hard on the knees of a man over 40, and the rate of injuries (twisted ankles, shin splints, etc.) among runners is alarmingly high. Besides, some studies show that you can get the same fitness benefits from walking a fifteen-minute mile as you do from running that mile. Swimming, as we've said, probably places the least amount of stress on your body and is an excellent aerobic and overall body conditioner.

Getting Started

If you are in good health you should be able to do all the things you were able to do at 30 or even 20. Of course, they may take you a little longer and tire you out a little more, but you can still do them. The most important thing to remember is to start slowly and choose an activity that fits your schedule, your energy level, and your attention span.

Read books. Check with health clubs, gyms, and the YMCA/YMHA. Look for skating rinks, gyms, pools, health clubs, and racquet clubs. Rent a bike, exercise to a video tape, or invest in a rowing machine. Exercising with a friend is often more enjoyable (it commits you to a program); but taking advantage of the solitude that exercise time gives you is wonderful, too. In other words, anything that works for you is great.

The idea is to make it as easy on yourself as possible, because in the long run, that's the only way you're going to keep it up.

The ideal exercise regimen works the entire body and combines three kinds of exercises: for flexibility, strength, and aerobic power. Each of them has certain benefits to an over-40 man, and aerobics is particularly important for cardiovascular fitness, but for all-around health you really need to combine all three. Whole books have been written about each of them, so of course, we can't hope to do anything but discuss the basics here. But the basics are a good place to start.

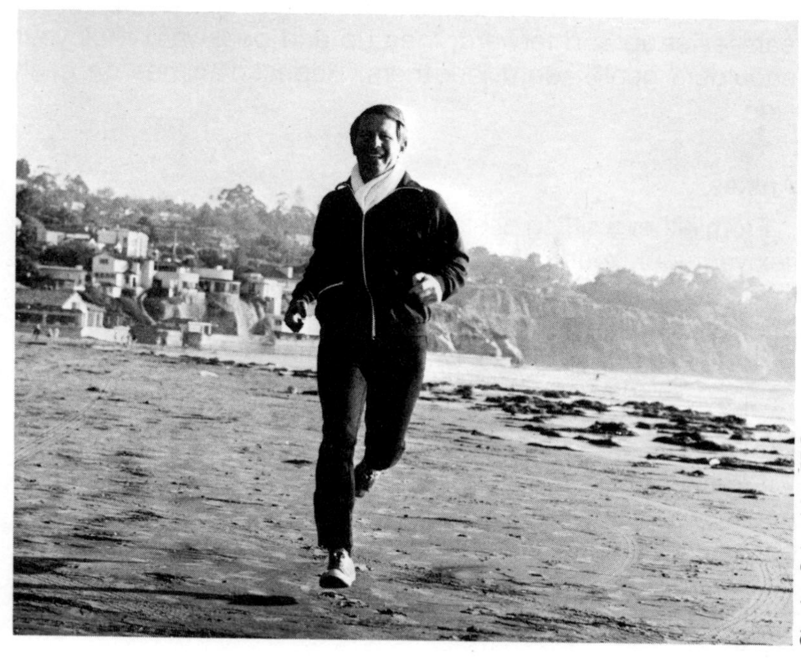

Charles Schneider, FPG

Stretching Exercises

Slow, sustained stretching lengthens and warms the muscles and keeps you from getting stiff, especially in the ankles, knees, back, neck, shoulders, and fingers. Stretching exercises also help relieve built-up daily tension. The following stretches may be used as a warm-up before aerobics.

Fingers

Extend your arms at your sides to shoulder level. Clench your hands into fists and then open your hands quickly, stretching your fingers and joints as much as possible. Repeat 20 times with each hand.

Shoulders

Sit up as straight as you can. Move your shoulders up to your ears—first up and forward, then up and backward. Roll your shoulders gently; don't jerk them. Repeat 10 times on each side.

Ankles

From either a sitting or standing position extend your leg and flex your foot. Your toes should be pointing up. Circle your foot to the left, pointing your toes down, until you've made a circle. Then circle to the right. Repeat 10 times in each direction. Then switch to the other foot.

Neck

From either a standing or sitting position relax your shoulders and let your arms hang at your sides. In a smooth motion (without bouncing) drop your head forward, then to the left, then backward, then to the front again. Repeat 10 times to the left, then 10 times to the right.

Back

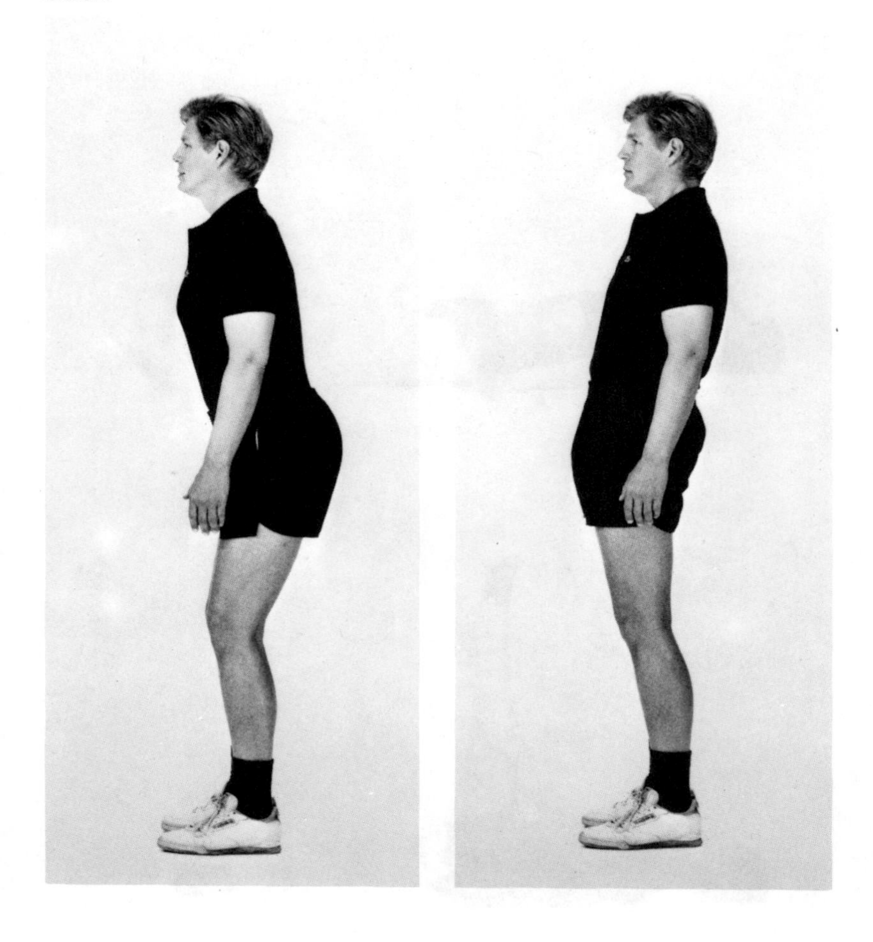

Stand up straight with your feet about 18 inches apart and your arms hanging at your sides. Arch your lower back and release your pelvis at the same time. Hold for 3 seconds. Then drop your buttocks and bring your back into line again, tilting your pelvis forward. Hold that for 3 seconds. Repeat 10 times.

Knees

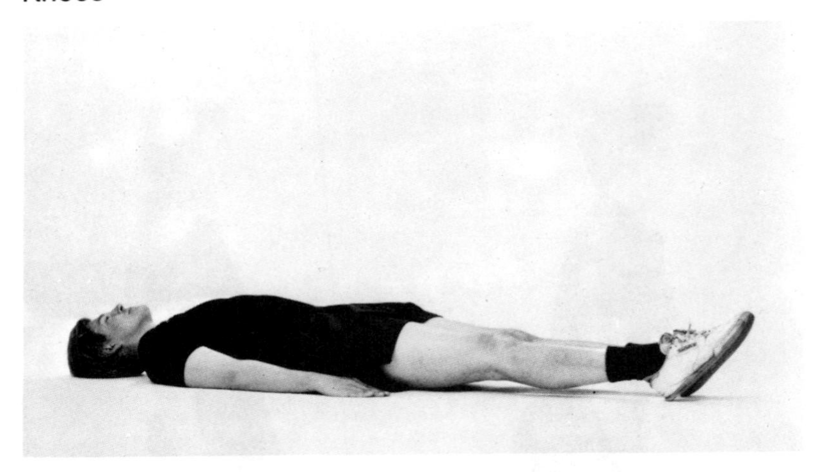

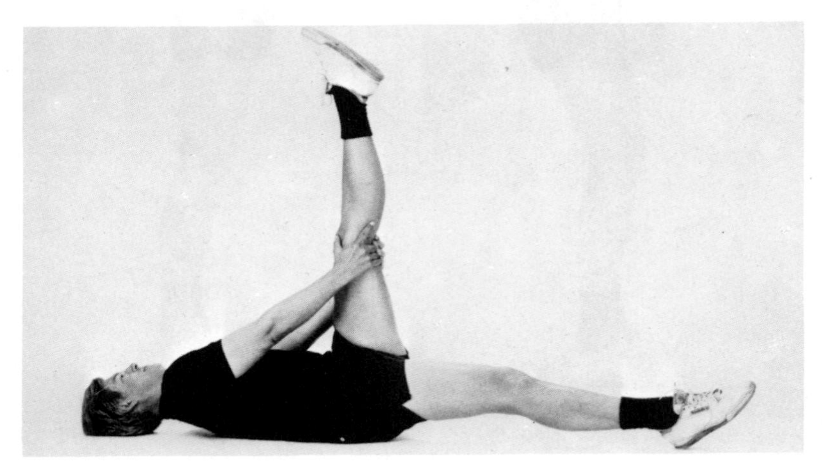

Lie on your back and extend your legs. Point your toes. With your hands clasped underneath your knee, pull your thigh toward your chest and press gently for a few seconds. Switch to the other leg. Repeat 15 times for each leg.

Groin

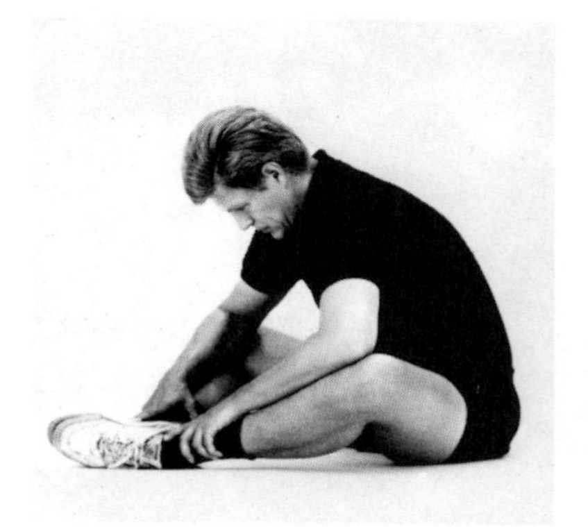

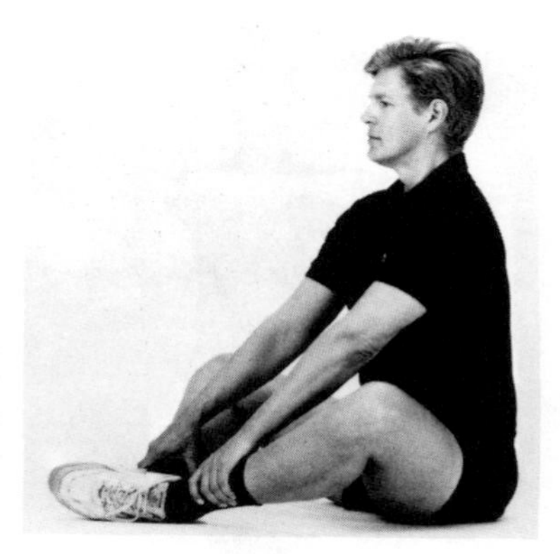

Sit on the floor with your knees out and the soles of your feet pressed together. Keep your back straight (if you have to lean forward, that's all right). Relax your shoulders and pull your abdomen in. Hold your ankles and gently press your knees as close to the floor as you can manage. Repeat 15 times.

Strengthening Exercises

When we think of exercises, these are usually what we have in mind—leg lifts, sit-ups, etc. In strengthening exercises specific muscles are subjected to repeated contractions, and the body's resistance plays a part in the muscle-building process.

Some men like to use weight machines for their strengthening exercises. If you want to give them a try, be sure to have someone teach you how to use them properly, and don't overdo it. And don't work out on machines two days in a row or more than three times a week. You may also decide to add free weights. Just build them up gradually.

Strengthening exercises give you a chance to concentrate on toning and firming up specific parts of your body. Some strengthening exercises that can help the problem areas most likely to need attention are described below. These are not too demanding, but don't forget—this is where you start.

Arms

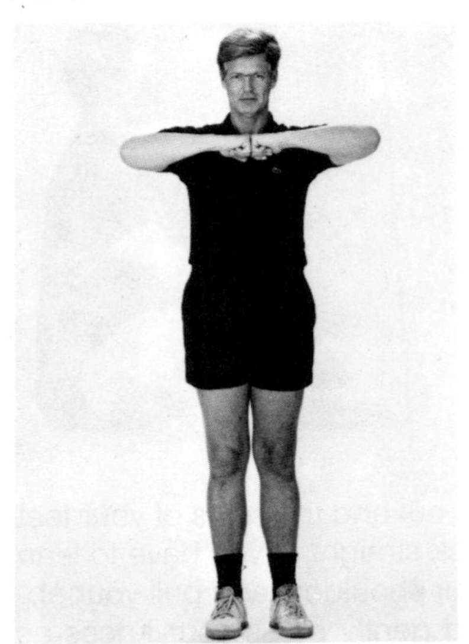

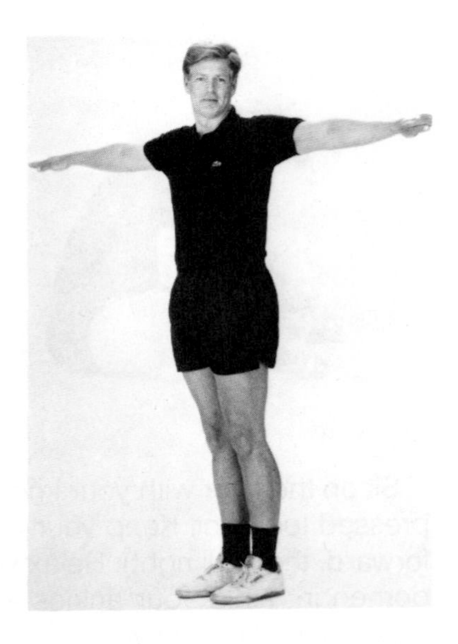

Stand with your legs together and your feet flat on the floor. Raise your bent elbows out to your sides, clenching your fists and holding them at chest level (as if you're imitating a clucking hen). Straighten your arms and stretch them out to your sides at shoulder level, unclenching your fists as you do so. Hold for 3 seconds. Clench your fists, bend your arms again, and hold them next to your chest again for a 3-second count. Repeat 15 times.

Chest

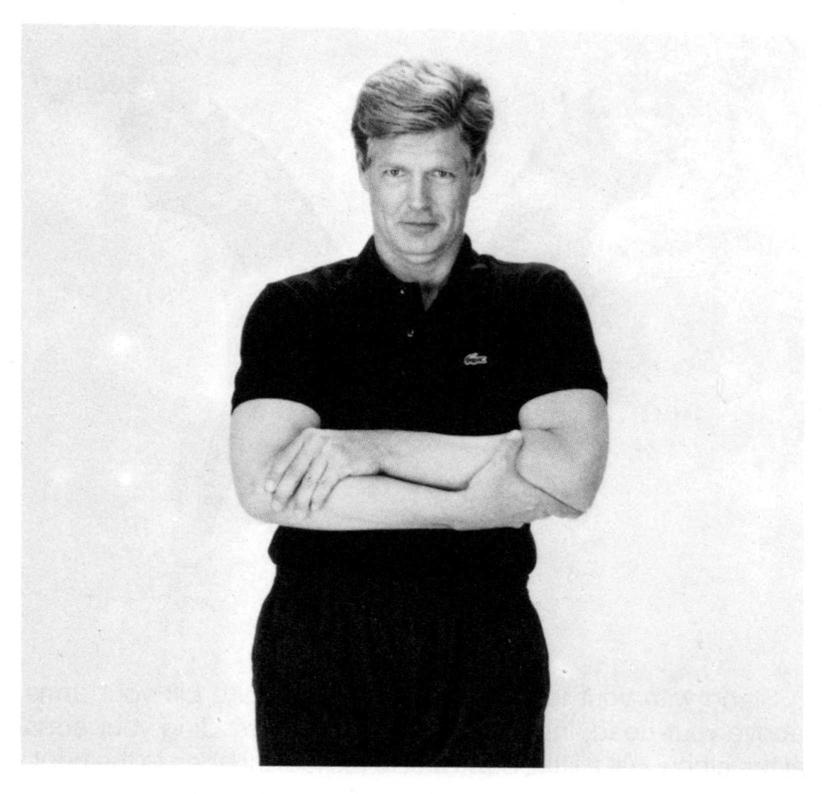

Stand with your legs together and your feet flat on the floor. Fold your arms by holding each forearm just below the elbow with the opposite hand. Without moving your hand up your arm, push hard toward your elbow. Repeat 20 times.

Waist

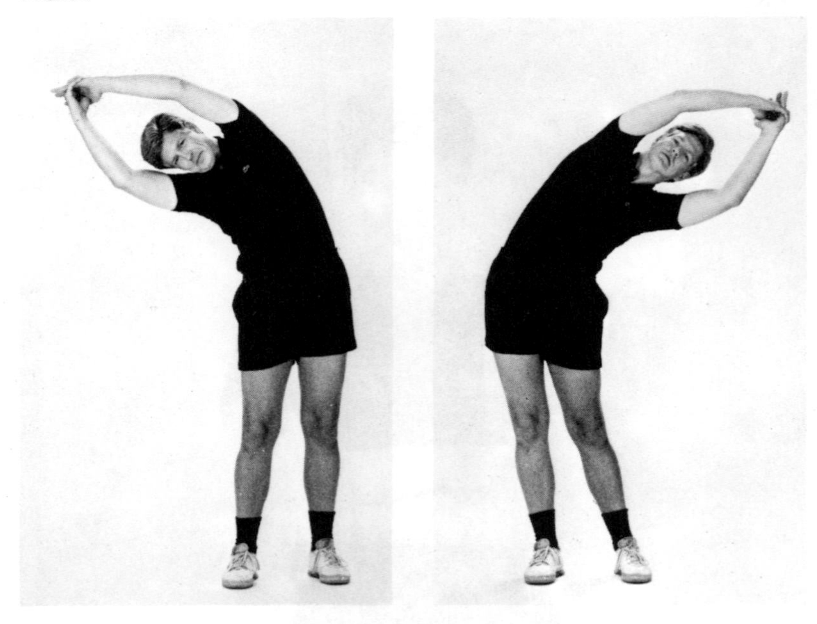

Stand with your legs about 12 inches apart. Lift your arms above your head, interlacing your fingers. Bending your arms at the elbow just a little, bend first to the left and then to the right. Don't let your torso move forward. Keep the motion gentle; don't bounce. Repeat 15 times.

Abdominals

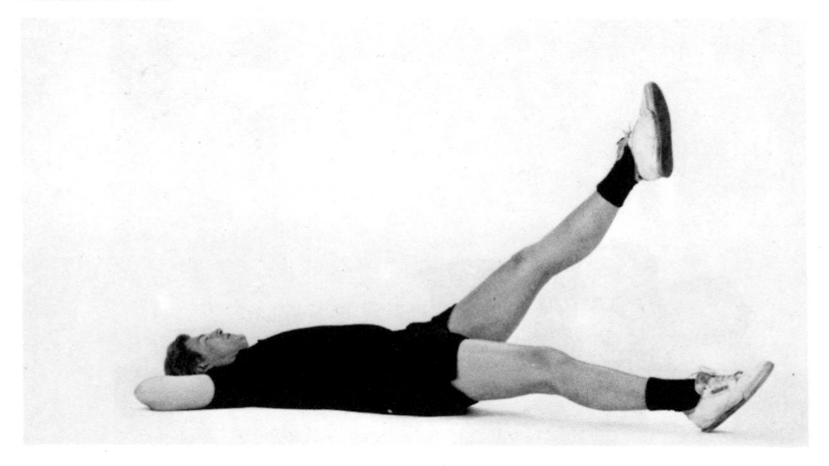

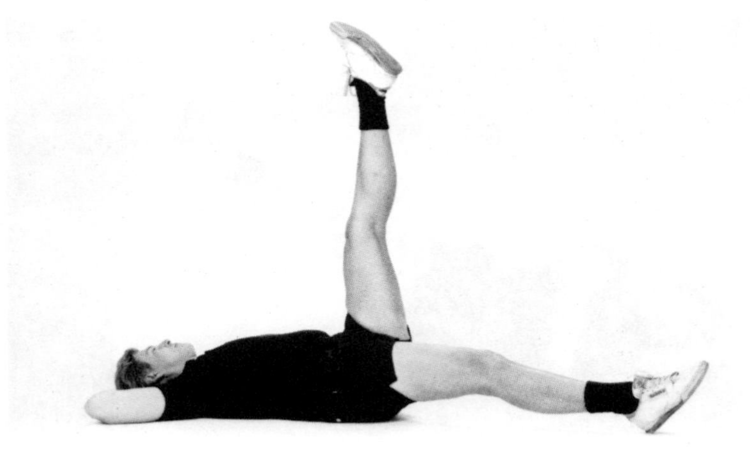

Lie flat on your back and put your arms under your head. Raise your right leg at a 45-degree angle and hold for 5 seconds. Then raise it all the way up and hold for 5 seconds. Lower your leg as slowly as you can. Switch legs. Repeat this 10 times with each leg.

Thighs

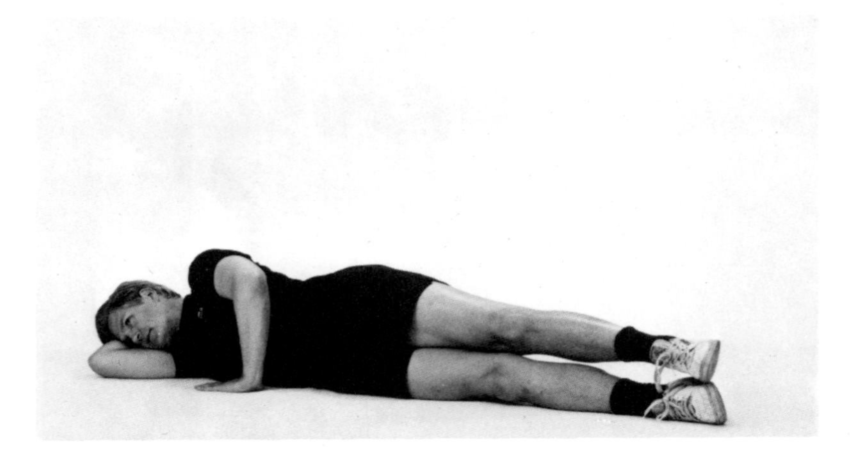

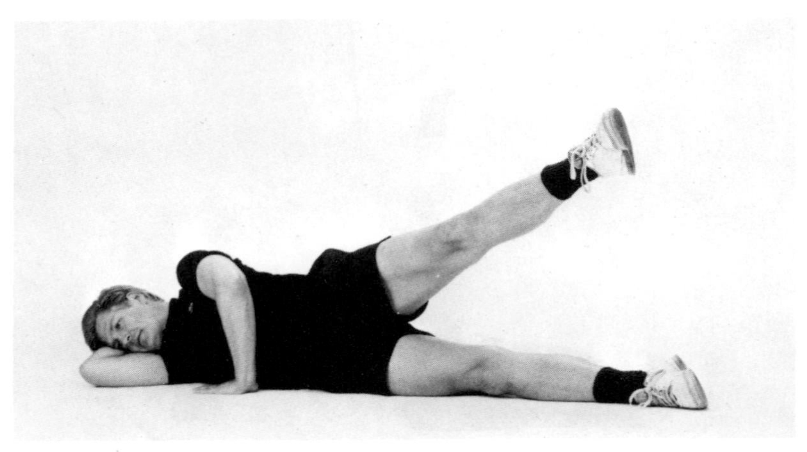

Lie on your side, supporting your head with one arm and balancing your body with the other (just below your chest). Raise the upper leg slowly, keeping your knees straight and your toes pointed. Bring your leg up as high as possible and hold for 5 seconds. Lower it as slowly as possible. Repeat 10 times, then do the exercise 10 times on the other side.

Buttocks

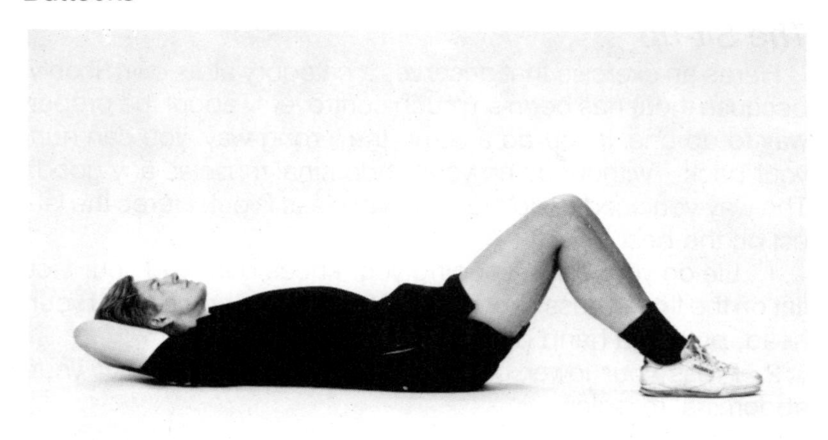

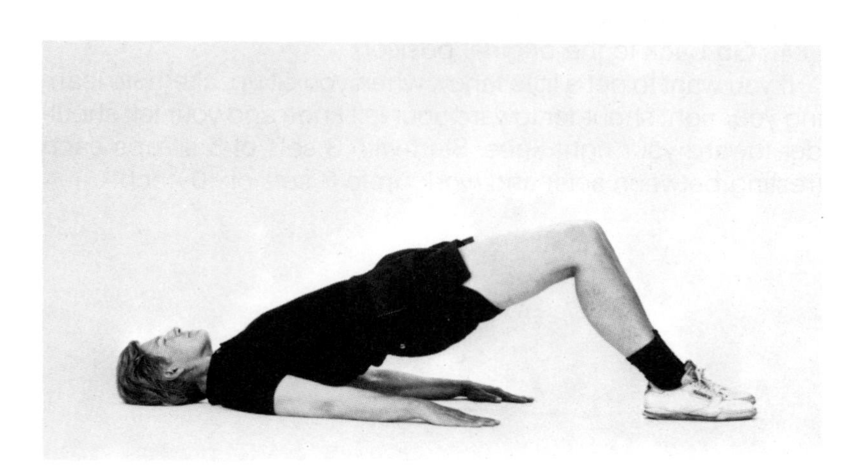

Lie on your back with your arms along your sides, palms on the floor. Bend your knees. Raise your bottom off the floor and tighten the muscles of your buttocks. Hold for 5 seconds. Repeat 12 times.

The Sit-up

Here's an exercise that deserves a category all its own, if only because there has been so much controversy about the proper way to do one. If you do a sit-up the wrong way, you can hurt your back—without doing your abdominal muscles any good. The way you used to do them in gym class is out. Here's the latest on the best sit-up:

1. Lie on your back, keeping your knees bent and your feet flat on the floor. Cross your arms all the way around behind your head, putting a hand on each shoulder.
2. Press your lower back into the floor and contract your abdominal muscles.
3. Bring your upper body up to a 30- to 45-degree angle, keeping your lower back on the floor at all times.
4. Go back to the original position.

If you want to get a little fancy, when you sit up, alternate leaning your right shoulder toward your left knee and your left shoulder toward your right knee. Start with 3 sets of 5 sit-ups each (resting between sets) and work up to 3 sets of 10 each.

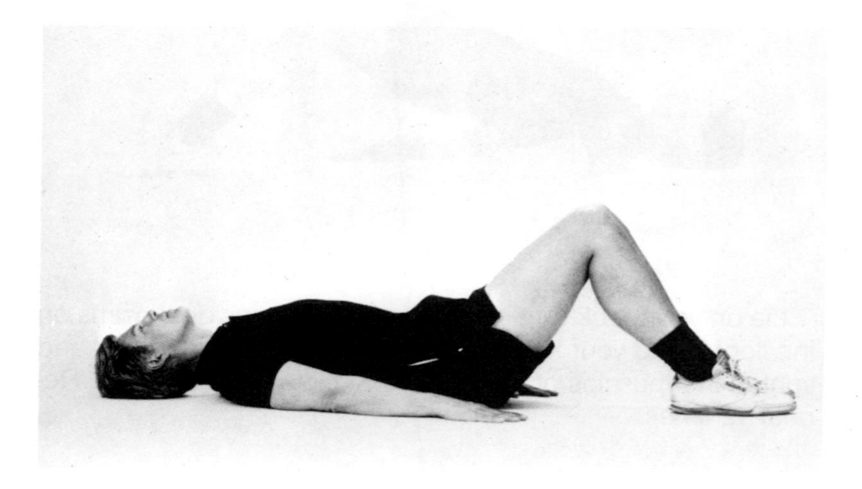

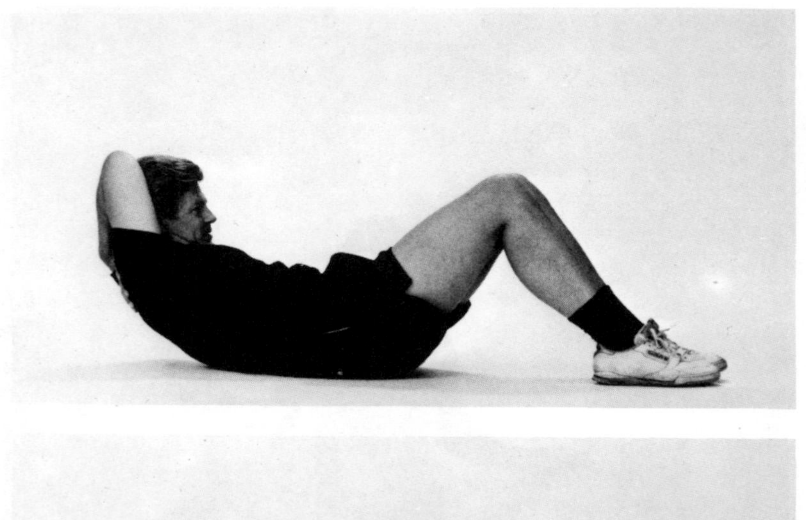

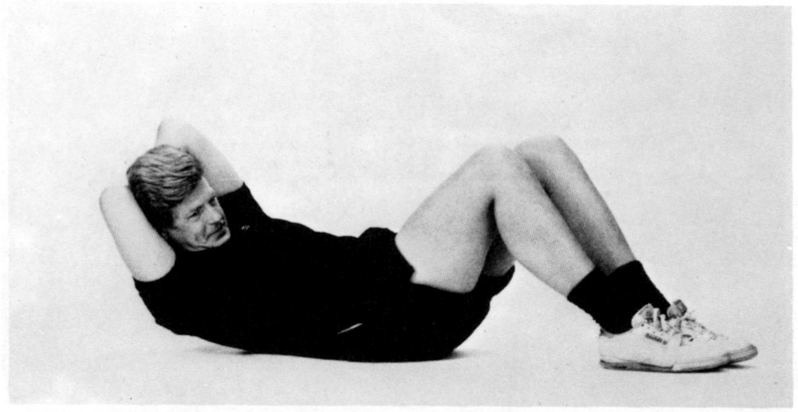

Exercise is not a panacea; there is no such thing. But combined with intelligent dietary choices and other self-care techniques, you can maintain your physique and level of activity far beyond what you might now consider possible. Again, see a physician before making any drastic increases in your physical-exertion level or any fundamental changes in your lifestyle. He'll probably tell you what you may already suspect: These are the best years of your life!

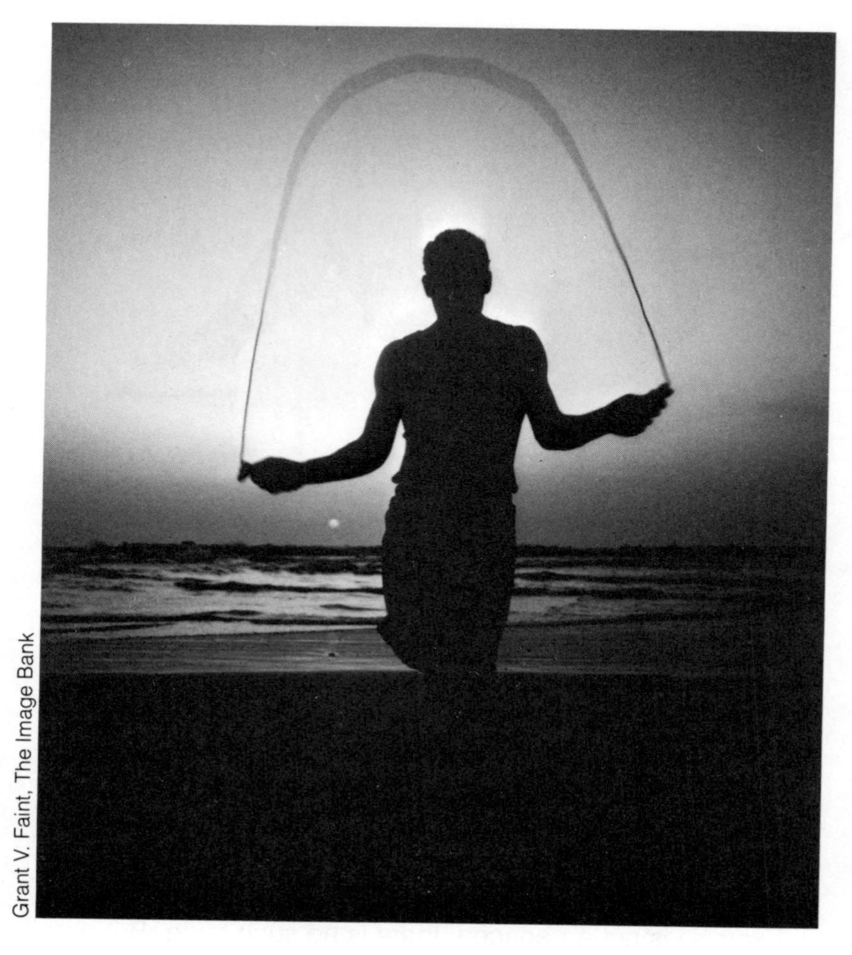

Grant V. Faint, The Image Bank

A jump rope can become part of your *portable* cardiovascular health program. Take it everywhere, but remember to wear "aerobic" sneakers and avoid jumping on hard surfaces.

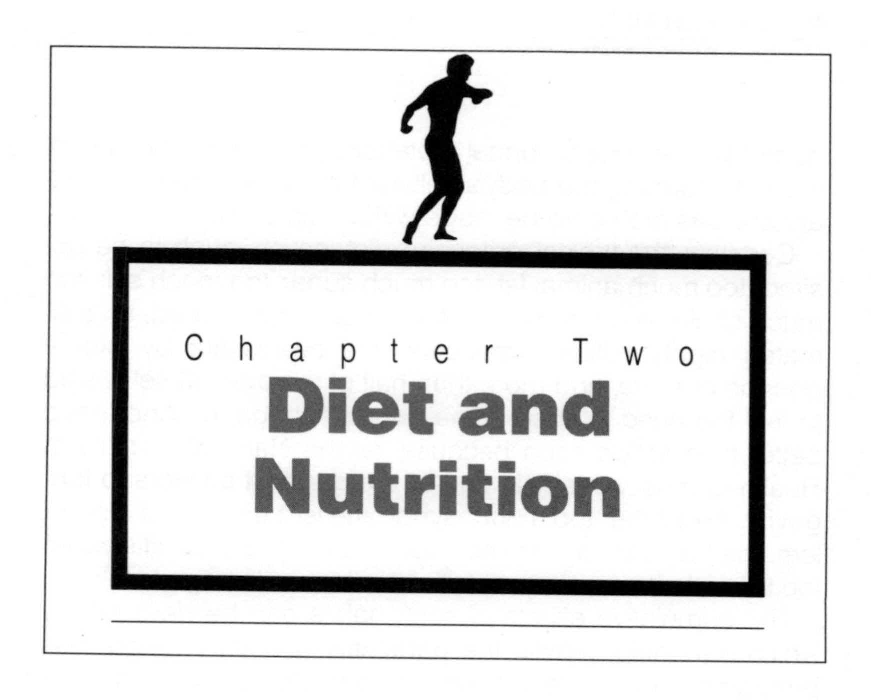

Chapter Two
Diet and Nutrition

We are what we eat, a fact of supreme importance throughout our lives but one that takes on far greater significance with age. A man entering or in his middle years faces the critical task of adopting sound eating practices that satisfy the particular needs of his lifestyle and also make good nutritional sense. It is a monumental task that will have an effect on virtually every aspect of his life and health.

Keeping the Body Young

Proper nutrition—or, rather, the lack of it—has been directly related to several age-related conditions, among them cardiovascular disease, periodontal disease, and cancer. Furthermore, the act of eating itself, says Sheldon Saul Hendler, author of *The Complete Guide to Anti-Aging Nutrients,* "increases the 'opportunities' for aging," meaning that we may often eat the "wrong" foods, may be exposed to potentially toxic food colorings and additives, or may suffer damage from "free radicals," which are unstable chemical compounds (some of them produced by the body's normal metabolic processes) capable of severely harming the body's cellular functioning. Clearly, dietary choices are not to be made without careful consideration.

Certainly, the typical American diet leaves much to be desired: too much animal fat, too much sugar, too much salt, too much cholesterol—too much food in general! Indeed, an estimated eighty million Americans are overweight by twenty pounds or more, and more than half of the over-40 set is said to feel the need to shed some excess "baggage." And they'd better take action soon because, as the National Institute of Health reports, **obesity is one of the greatest barriers to longevity.** And if the "too much" syndrome isn't enough of a problem, the "too little" syndrome—too little exercise, too little water, too little attention paid to nutrition—causes damage too.

The cumulative effects of such habits can be devastating, which may help explain the popularity of instant weight-loss programs. The trouble is, these fad diets are not only ineffective over the long run, but worse, they are often damaging to the body—especially the over-50 body—since most weight loss usually occurs not through burning off excess fat but through the loss of water and active tissue.

The key point to remember is that losing weight is not the ultimate goal: Rather, it is to arrive at the proper balance between caloric intake and exercise so as to maintain your ideal weight.

The following table, adapted from the Metropolitan Life Insurance charts, shows the ideal height and weight for men.

So how does a man over 40 attain or maintain these weight levels and improve his chances of living longer? First determine how many calories you should consume daily (multiply your weight, or desired weight, by 15, to find out how many calories you can consume for a fairly low activity level), then adhere to the following guidelines:

- **Reduce your intake of sugar**—both in refined form and as it appears in processed foods. Check labels for sucrose, glucose, corn syrup, and dextrose. Despite that fact that

	Weight in Pounds		
Height	Small frame	Medium frame	Large frame
5′1″	112–120	118–129	126–141
5′2″	115–123	121–133	129–144
5′3″	118–126	124–136	132–148
5′4″	121–129	127–139	135–152
5′5″	124–133	130–143	138–156
5′6″	128–137	134–137	142–161
5′7″	132–141	138–152	147–166
5′8″	136–145	142–156	151–170
5′9″	140–150	146–160	155–174
5′10″	144–154	150–165	159–179
5′11″	148–158	154–170	164–184
6′	152–162	158–175	169–189
6′1″	156–167	162–180	173–194
6′2″	160–171	167–185	178–199
6′3″	164–175	172–190	182–204

sugar has been shown to contribute to tooth decay, adult onset diabetes, hypertension, heart disease, and liver and adrenal problems, the average American has what appears to be an unquenchable sweet tooth, consuming sugar at a rate of about one teaspoon *every* 35 minutes *every* day of the year!

- **Reduce your intake of salt.** Salt is the body's main source of sodium, which is needed to regulate body fluids. It is also America's second most popular food additive, after sugar, and as with sugar the average American consumes too much—about twice the recommended daily allotment of one half to one and a half teaspoons. While it has not been proved that excess sodium causes high blood pres-

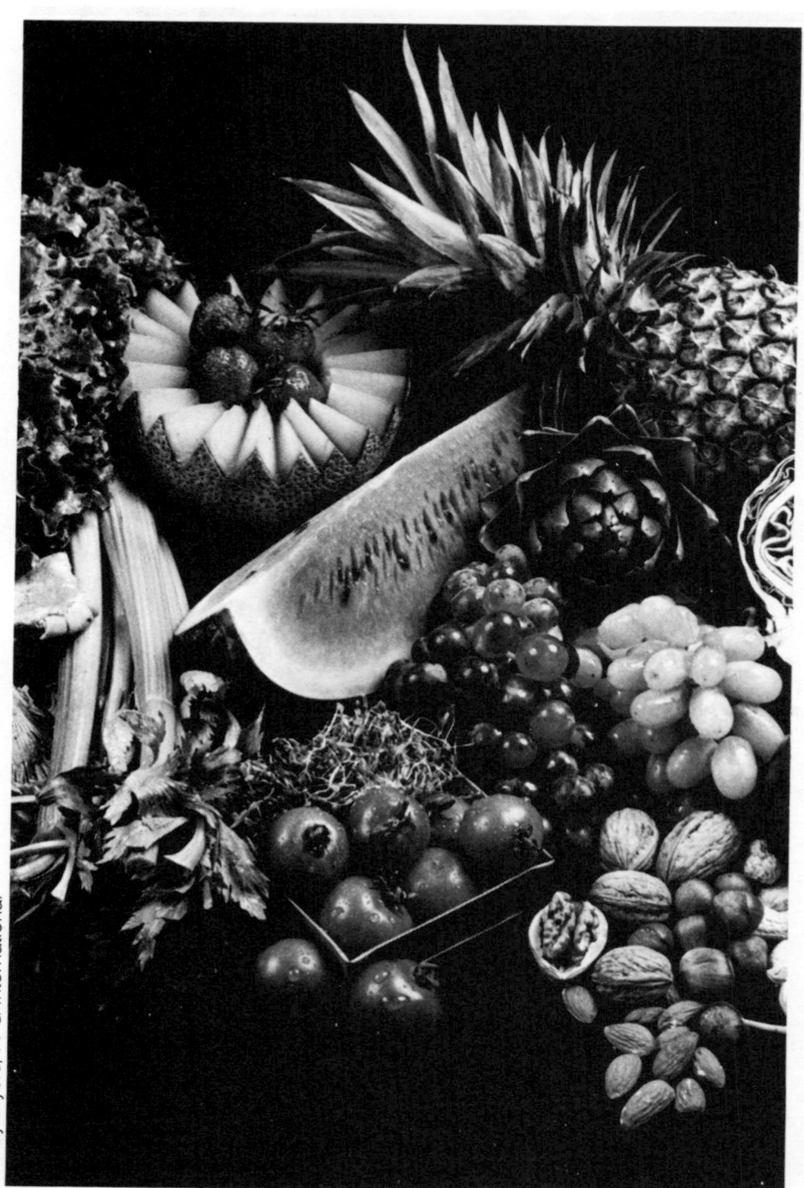

Jeffrey Myers, FPG International

sure or that maintaining a low level of sodium consumption can prevent hypertension from occurring, all doctors agree that *a low-sodium diet can reduce blood pressure in patients who already have high blood pressure.* Furthermore, studies of countries with low-sodium diets show hardly any incidence of high blood pressure. Because this appears to lend significant support to the idea that diets low in sodium can have a preventive effect, the Food and Nutrition Board of the National Academy of Sciences National Research Council has recommended low-sodium diets not just for hypertensives but for the general public as well. You can reduce your salt intake by cooking with spices and herbs rather than salt, avoiding processed or canned foods (salt is an often-used and inexpensive taste enhancer and preservative), keeping your saltshaker in an out-of-the-way-place (the inconvenience of retrieving it will help you break the habit), and reading labels carefully—even those marked "low sodium," "no salt added," etc. And remember: You'll most likely get your daily requirement of sodium simply by sticking to a well-balanced diet.

- **Reduce your intake of cholesterol,** which is said to be the number-one risk factor for cardiovascular disease. Cholesterol is found in eggs, meat, dairy products, and, to a lesser extent, poultry and fish. Thus you should try to eat "lean" meats and fish and chicken without the skin. And the simple fact is that we eat too much cholesterol. According to Jane Brody's *The New York Times Guide to Personal Health,* "To meet basic nutritional needs we need to eat only one tablespoon of a polyunsaturated oil each day . . . the average American adult eats six to eight times this amount . . . making fat a major source of nutritionally empty calories for millions of Americans." Read the section below called "Food for a Healthy Heart" and also Chapter One to see how exercise can help combat high levels of blood cholesterol.

- **Reduce the percentage of your total caloric intake that is derived from saturated fats (animal fats).** The typical American diet contains at least 40 percent fat (mostly animal fat): over twice the amount it should. Try to limit fat intake to 15 or 20 percent of the polyunsaturated variety, found in nuts, seeds, and vegetable oils. Fat is not only unhealthy but causes fatigue by preventing oxygen-carrying red blood cells from getting to muscles and other tissues.
- **Avoid simple and refined carbohydrates; concentrate instead on complex carbohydrates.** Simple/refined carbohydrates include: all sugars and refined flour found in packaged mixes. Complex carbohydrates—fibers and starches—include: rice, pasta, legumes, nuts, seeds, whole-grain bread, and fruits and vegetables. The typical American diet contains 40 percent carbohydrates, but it should contain 65 to 70 percent *complex* carbohydrates. The high percentage of complex carbohydrates is warranted for several reasons: Complex carbohydrates are the body's primary source of energy; they comprise the only category of food with no established connection to any of the major "killer" diseases; they produce a "full" sensation before too many calories are consumed (thus aiding weight loss); and—contrary to popular belief—they are not fattening but instead contain little fat and cholesterol and many nutrients.
- **Avoid consuming too much protein, particularly too many animal proteins,** which bring with them animal fat. Instead, consider non-animal sources of protein such as tofu, nuts, and legumes.
- **Avoid food additives and food colorings,** whose links to cancer and other ailments are always under review.
- **Avoid nitrite-cured or smoked foods,** which may increase a man's risk of developing cancer in the stomach or esophagus.

- **Avoid food that has been broiled, fried, or grilled.** Opt instead for stewed, sautéed, poached, or baked foods. In the case of meat, fish, or poultry the former methods create browned or charred parts of food that contain substances that may be carcinogenic.
- **Limit your consumption of alcohol.** Besides acting as a depressant and causing liver damage alcohol can both raise and lower blood pressure, so moderation is in order. It's also filled with empty calories and depletes the body of vitamin C, many of the B vitamins, and calcium, magnesium, potassium and zinc.
- **Limit your intake of caffeine,** found in coffee, teas, chocolate, colas, and even aspirin. While the link of caffeine to heart attacks is a subject of debate, it definitely affects your nervous system. It constricts your blood vessels and stimulates your adrenal glands. It depletes your body of vitamin C, calcium, potassium, and zinc. (*Warning:* The caffeine-removing chemicals in decaffeinated coffee can be harmful.)
- **Don't smoke.** If you still smoke, it bears repeating that smoking has been linked to lung cancer, cardiovascular disease, chronic bronchitis, and emphysema. If you don't smoke, don't start.
- **Eat a variety of foods from the major food groupings:** milk, meat, grains, and fruits and vegetables.
- **Eat more fiber,** which is found in fruits, vegetables, whole grains, and beans. Fiber contains little fat and few calories and at the same time is very filling—so filling, in fact, that it produces a "full" feeling that reduces the tendency to overeat. Some evidence has also shown that fiber may lower blood pressure, prevent diabetes, and offer protection against colon cancer. It is thought that most Americans can safely increase their intake of dietary fiber. However, if you suffer from any gastrointestinal conditions such as colitis or ileitis, you should first get your physician

to set a proper level of fiber consumption for you. Fiber is a form of "roughage" that improves digestive functions generally but can aggravate any abnormalities or even cause a condition in which the sigmoid colon becomes twisted and enlarged. Increased flatulence and bloating are other side effects of increased fiber intake, but these are temporary conditions and should wear off once your body becomes used to the presence of this new substance.

- **Drink lots of water,** anywhere from five to eight glasses a day. Water is a vital fluid that cleanses the body of toxins and aids in circulation.
- **Eat only when you are hungry and only as much as you need to feel satisfied.** Overeating induces fatigue and sluggishness.
- **Eat breakfast.** (You've always suspected as much, haven't you?) Giving yourself a shot of energy in the morning (eating breakfast raises your blood-sugar level, which in turn sparks body and brain activity) is vitally important for elevating both your productivity and your disposition. One study that tracked 7,000 people over ten years showed that skipping breakfast was one of several factors that, when taken together, increased the likelihood that a man would not live to his full life expectancy.
- **Eat your largest meal in the middle of the day and try not to eat too much shortly before your bedtime.** This allows your body to use the nutrients you feed it more effectively. A dinner consisting mostly of carbohydrates—such as pasta—will help you sleep.
- **Eat vitamin-A-containing vegetables** such as broccoli, cauliflower, brussels sprouts, and cabbage and vitamin-C-laden fruits such as cantaloupe, oranges, strawberries, and grapefruit, which have all been shown to decrease the incidence of various cancers (stomach, esophagus, and colon). These foods should be added liberally to your diet.

- **Be smart about vitamin and mineral supplements.** Eating a variety of foods that will fulfill the recommended daily dietary allowances is still the best way to give your body what it needs, but some form of supplement is often deemed necessary. Luckily, supplements taken in moderation and with specific goals in mind appear capable of having positive effects on counteracting cancer, heart disease, and most other age-related malfunctions. And the medical profession may finally be "coming around" to their widespread use, so you might want to seek out the advice of a doctor to help you decide which supplements and in what amounts would serve you best. (See the Vitamin/Mineral Chart on pages 54–55.)
- **Include these "superfoods" in your diet** (cited by *Prevention* magazine):

amaranth
bananas
beans
bran
cabbage-family vegetables (including broccoli, cauliflower, and brussels sprouts)
carrots
citrus fruits
fish (salmon and mackerel only)
herbs and spices
leafy green vegetables (such as kale and spinach)
liver
melons
nuts
oysters (not raw)
peppers
poultry
seeds
soup
soybeans
sprouts
sweet potatoes
wheat germ
whole grains
yogurt

Food for a Healthy Heart

If you follow the nutritional suggestions above you'll be well on your way to combating the dietary factors that contribute to cardiovascular disease. But there are some additional facts to keep in mind.

Cholesterol damages the heart by gathering along the walls of the blood vessels, gradually narrowing the arteries and restricting the flow of blood. Not everyone realizes that cholesterol is also manufactured by the body—in the liver—and that a certain amount of it is necessary early in life to create cell membranes and to contribute to bone development and the production of sex hormones. Unfortunately, often too much of it remains in the body—mostly through diet—after it has performed its vital functions. Many researchers feel that after the first six months of life we no longer need cholesterol in our diet.

The American diet is in many ways to blame. The average American man has about 210 to 220 milligrams of cholesterol per 100 milliliters of blood. This is very close to the danger zone —260 milligrams—that, according to the Framingham Heart Study, makes a man *three times* more likely to experience cardiovascular disease. While the Japanese exhibit very little heart trouble, owing to their generally low cholesterol diet, Japanese immigrants to this country who adopt the basic American diet show increased incidence of cardiovascular trouble.

Certain minerals—selenium, magnesium, and potassium— have been shown to play a role in keeping the heart working well. Selenium, in particular, has generated considerable excitement because of its apparent ability to act against heart disease. Evidence of its powers was gathered in a study conducted in the southeastern United States, a region known as the "stroke belt" because it has the country's highest stroke rate as well as a very high incidence of heart disease. Researchers, who suspected that the low selenium levels in the region's soil might have something to do with these figures, reported that selenium supplements to the diet showed promising results in reducing the occurrence of heart disease and stroke. It has also been demonstrated that selenium has the ability to act against cancer. Says the National Academy of Sciences: "A large accumulation of evidence indicates that supplementation of the diet or drinking water with selenium protects against tumors in-

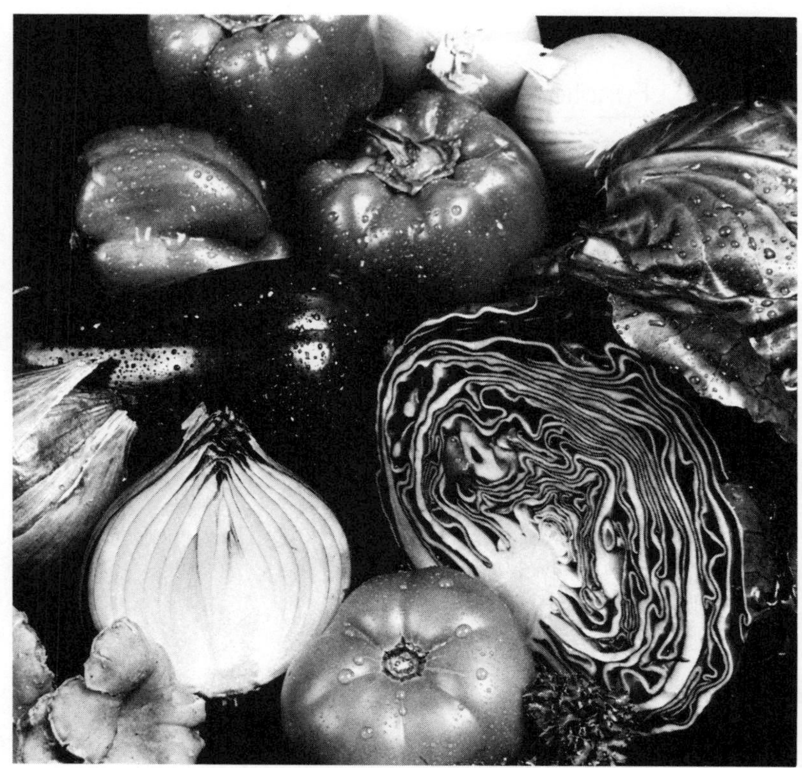

Jeffrey Myers, FPG International

duced by a variety of chemical carcinogens and at least one viral agent . . ." Selenium is found in grains, fish, cabbage, broccoli, onions, radishes, mushrooms, and organ meats. *Note: Selenium is highly toxic if taken in excess; fortunately, it appears that only small doses of this mineral are needed for it to be effective.*

Vitamin	Functions	RDA	Good Sources
A	Indispensable for healthy skin, hair, and eyes. Good for the bones and teeth and for keeping the mucus membranes moist.	5,000 IU	eggs, milk, liver, butter, cheese, and all kinds of fruits and vegetables
E	Good for the skin. It helps to form muscles and red blood cells, and it maintains good circulation.	30 IU	vegetable oil and shortening, whole grains, leafy green vegetables, and liver
C	Also called ascorbic acid, it forms and maintains collagen, helps to maintain teeth, bones, and small blood vessels, and may stimulate the immune system. (The last is why vitamin C is touted as being effective against the common cold and even cancer.)	60 mg	citrus fruits, strawberries, dark-green vegetables, cabbage, tomatoes, sweet potatoes, and melons
D	Works with minerals to keep your bones and teeth healthy. Assists in the absorption of calcium and phosphorus.	400 IU	milk, fish, egg yolks, liver, butter, and sunlight
THE B's	These are indispensable for healthy skin, nervous system, and an active metabolism. Aid in the formation of red blood cells.		grains, dried beans and peas, legumes, dairy products, eggs, meat, dark-green vegetables, and fish
Thiamine (B_1)		1.5 mg	
Riboflavin (B_2)		1.7 mg	
Niacin (B_3)	These are the most important B vitamins for a man in his forties.	20 mg	

Pantothenic Acid (B_5)		10 mg	
Pyridoxine (B_6)		2 mg	
Folic Acid		.5 mg	

Mineral

Calcium	Vital for the health of your bones. Assists normal blood clotting and heart functions.	800–1,000 mg	milk, cheese, dark-green vegetables, and soybeans
Iron	Keeps the blood supplied with oxygen.	20 mg	meat, organ meats (such as liver), poultry, egg yolks, dried beans, grains, cereals, sunflower seeds, garbanzos
Zinc	Heals the skin, builds proteins in the body, and helps metabolism. Also intensifies action and absorption of other minerals.	15 mg	chicken, eggs, fish, yogurt, milk, wheat germ, bran, tofu, raisins, spinach, parsley, and mushrooms
Phosphorus	Essential for healthy bones, tissues, and teeth.	1,000 mg	eggs, fish, poultry, meat, dairy products, and dried peas and beans
Magnesium	Builds bones. Maintains heart arteries and is good for nerves and muscles.	400 mg	meat, seafood, green vegetables, and dairy products
Potassium	Important for the nerves and muscles. Regulates water balance in cells and helps keep blood pressure stable.	1,800–5,000 mg	bananas, baked potatoes, sunflower seeds, raisins, dates, and garbanzo beans

Magnesium is found in dairy products, green vegetables, and seafood; deficiencies of this mineral may foster conditions that lead to the formation of dangerous blood clots in the arteries. Potassium, found in bananas, fish such as salmon, flounder, and sardines, squash, potatoes, and chicken, has been called a "natural high blood pressure preventive" because it eases the arterial stress associated with high sodium levels in the bloodstream.

The fatty acid found in oily fish is good for the heart. Eicosapentanoic acid (EPA), the miracle ingredient found in salmon, mackerel, tuna, herring, trout, and sable, lowers blood pressure, decreases triglycerides, and reduces clotting. The Eskimos, who have a low incidence of heart disease, apparently owe their good health to the EPA found in whale and seal meat. Eating foods with EPA even once or twice a week may decrease your risk of heart attack.

Nutritionists

You might also want to consult a nutritionist or registered dietician, though these are best brought into the picture only if you have a very specific need. According to Susan Calvert Finn, the national chairperson of public relations for the American Dietetic Association and herself a specialist in nutrition, "Most of us don't require the services of a nutritionist at most times in our lives. The rule of thumb is that you probably need such services only if you have been diagnosed as having a medical or nutritional condition in which dietary factors play a part."

Since nutritionists do not need to be licensed, there are a good many questionable practitioners, and finding a respectable one will probably take a little work—for instance, asking your doctor or local medical society for a referral. You may be better off with a registered dietician who has gone through rigorous training, including four years of schooling, an internship, and passing an exam given by the ADA. Again, your doctor and local medical professionals are your best sources of information. The ADA at 430 North Michigan Avenue, Chicago, Illinois 60601, can also answer your questions.

For further discussion of nutrition in general, consult *Jane Brody's Nutrition Book, Diet for a Small Planet* by Frances Moore Lapple, *Nutrition for the Prime of Your Life* by Annette Naton and Jo-Anne Heslin, and *The Complete Guide to Anti-Aging Nutrients* by Sheldon Saul Hendler.

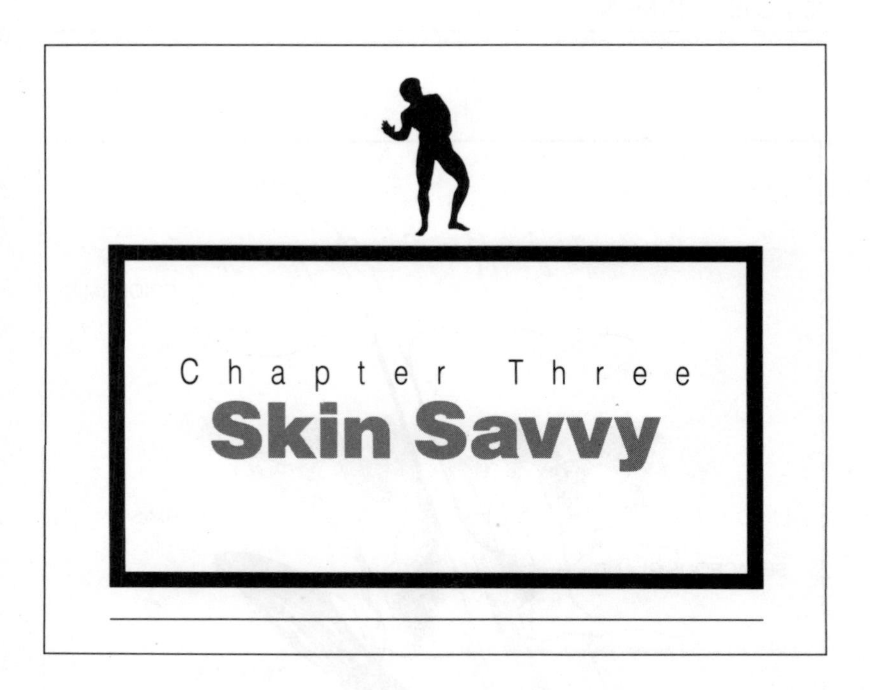

Chapter Three
Skin Savvy

At first glance, the print advertisement looks fairly typical for the grooming and cosmetics industry. Pictured is a medicine chest stocked with familiar items: pills, scissors, bandages, a razor, a comb, a toothbrush . . .The highlighted items, however, are the skin-care products—scruffing lotion, shaving cream, clean-scalp shampoo, moisturizer, etc. The copy attests to the products' powers, and, overall, the picture is both aesthetically pleasing and effective—you want to buy these products. Again, there is nothing out of the ordinary—except for one thing: The skin-care supplies being offered are for *men*.

Clinique introduced its skin-care system for men in 1976—a pioneer move, considering that at that time, for most men, skin care constituted a quick lathering up with whatever soap was in the dish and a slapping-on of some alcohol-based aftershave lotion. What was then hardly an afterthought is now, a decade later, a $45 million industry. Now the field is crowded and men —from college to middle age—are fast building up an interest in toiletries and skin-care products.

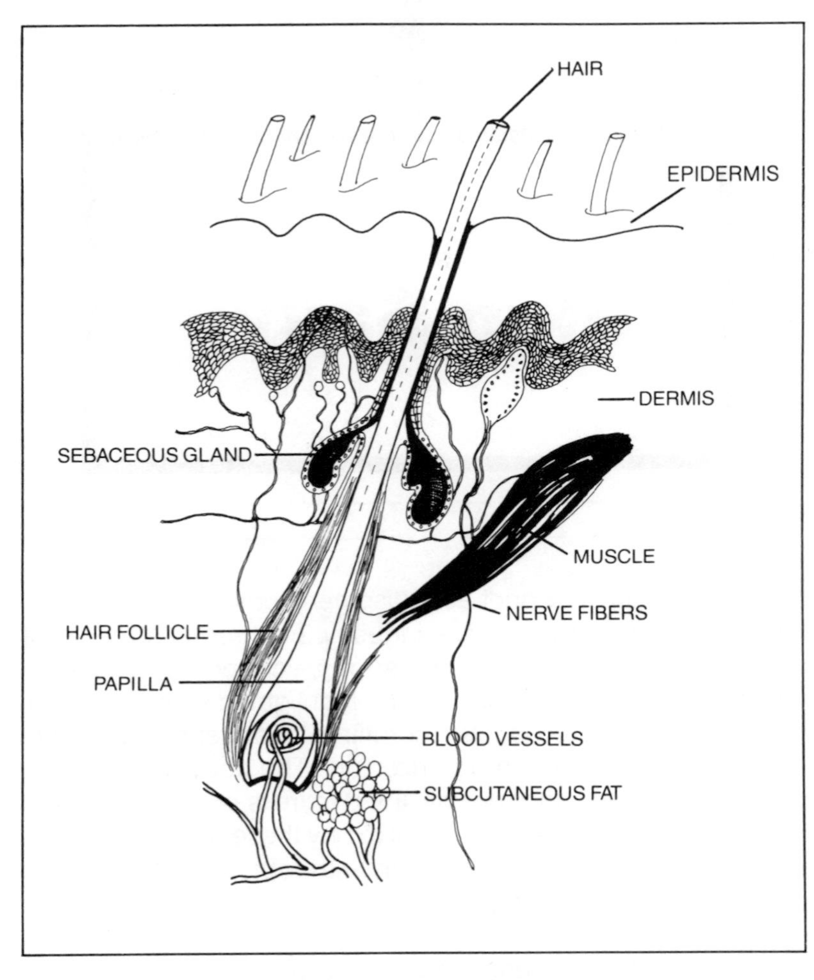

Cross Section of Skin

The new skin awareness among men of all ages is an obvious outgrowth of the nationwide fitness craze. It has been accompanied by what *Harper's Bazaar* has called a "new idea of masculinity." The Marlboro man's craggy face has fallen out of favor and been replaced by a smoother, more vital-looking appearance. This is good news for the man over 40, whose skin is beginning to show signs of age, because it means that doctors, scientists, and corporations are spending more time and money on developing new skin-care products for men and are trying to understand why the skin ages in the first place.

Skin: the Largest Organ in the Body

Skin's main functions are to protect the internal organs, to retain the proper amount of moisture in the body, and to regulate the body's temperature. But it is also a sophisticated sensory organ, consisting of two principal layers: the *epidermis,* or outer layer, and the *dermis,* or inner layer. Constantly renewing itself, the epidermis is penetrated by numerous nerve endings and consists of fifteen to twenty layers of cells that are continuously multiplying, working their way toward the surface, and dying—at which point they are shed. The dermis is made up of connective tissue fibers, nerve endings, hair follicles, and skin glands; blood and lymphatic vessels and nerves pass through it. The connective tissue is actually composed of a network of collagen and elastin fibers that weave through the dermis, forming a support system. *It is these fibers that give skin its strength and elasticity, and it is these fibers that deteriorate with age.*

According to skin-care expert Georgette Klinger, most people's skin ages in the same way:

- The collagen and elastin fibers stiffen, causing the skin to sag and lose much of its natural elasticity.
- The oil glands in the outer layer of the skin produce less oil (called sebum), while at the same time the inner layer becomes less able to retain water.
- The rate at which the skin cells regenerate slows down,

less collagen and elastin are produced, and tiny capillaries beneath the skin begin to close off.

In addition to these biochemical changes, by age 40 skin begins showing signs of its exposure to environmental and lifestyle factors, which include ultraviolet rays from the sun (skin's number-one enemy and the cause of 90 percent of all cases of skin cancer), smoking (which decreases the blood supply to the skin), alcohol (which dehydrates the skin), pollution, lack of exercise, poor nutrition, and even the force of gravity.

Facial expressions—frowns, smiles, grimaces—form creases that are likely to create lines and wrinkles because of the skin's diminished resiliency and ability to "bounce back" into shape. Genetics also comes into play—one can inherit a tendency toward broken capillaries, age spots, and bags and circles under the eyes.

Fortunately, most of the factors influencing the skin's health are within our control (genetics being the obvious exception—although there are "corrective" procedures for these problems as well). Since a man over 40 does not undergo abrupt hormonal changes at midlife (as does a woman passing into menopause) and has naturally thicker skin to begin with, he will most likely look younger than a woman of the same age. And, of course, wrinkles are not necessarily considered a detriment to a man's handsomeness. Such natural advantages are fine, of course, but they are not enough. As with most areas of personal health, asserting some control is the preferred modus operandi.

What's Your Skin Type?

The first step in taking control of your skin care is to identify your skin type. According to *Lia Schorr's Skin Care Guide for Men,* "Most men can handily rattle off vital statistics like their height, their weight. . . but they have no idea whether their skin . . . is dry, oily, or in between. This lack of knowledge. . . leads to needless rashes, allergies, blemishes, and even permanent

What's Your Skin Type?

Pore Size	Appearance	Skin Type
Large	Shiny, acne-prone, slightly bumpy texture, tans easily	Oily
Small	Smooth even texture, no shine, tans slowly	Normal
Very Small	Dull color, often chapped or flaky, freckles/burns easily	Dry

scars. . ." Once you know your skin type , you can go on to the next step: selecting the proper cleansing agent.

Washing

"Superfatted" soaps are best for men with dry skin, while conventional soaps are fine for those with oily skin. Men with sensitive skin—you qualify for this category if you are troubled to an inordinate degree by acne, shaving, or rashes—should not wash with deodorant soaps, the special ingredients of which increase the chance that some kind of irritation will occur. (Actually, even men with normal skin shouldn't wash with deodorant soaps!)

While washing your face (twice a day), the actual cleansing motion should be gentle. Although the objective is to rid the skin of sweat, bacteria, dead skin cells, and dirt, if you scrub too vigorously you will strip away vital oils or even cells that are not ready to be sloughed off. Don't use a washcloth—it's harsh on your skin and may harbor germs. It's also best not to wash with extremely hot or extremely cold water, despite what you may have heard about the latter's ability to close pores and create tighter, smoother-looking skin. Temperature extremes actually

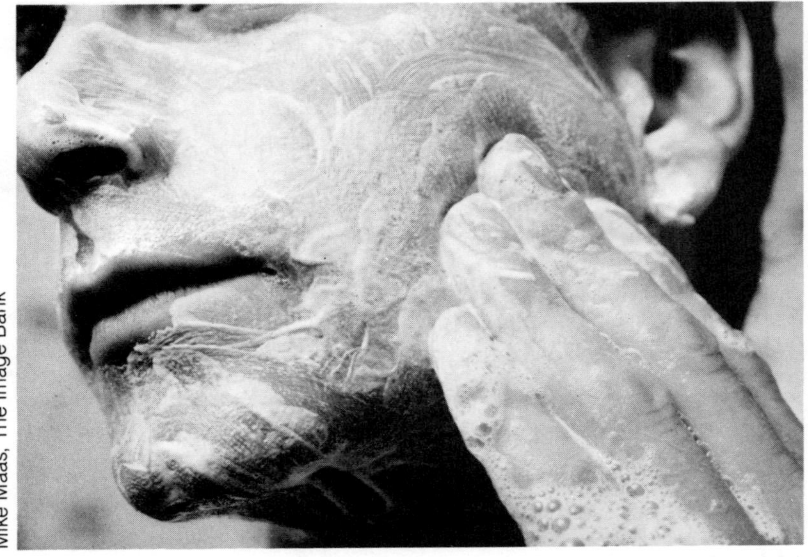

Mike Maas, The Image Bank

place stress on the skin, and hot water robs the skin of moisture. Most importantly, make sure you rinse well—it's the soap residue that dries out skin.

Toners, Refreshers, and Astringents

Products labeled toners, refreshers, or astringents deep-cleanse your skin. Astringents, which usually contain alcohol, should only be used by those with oily skin since they strip off natural oil—as well as dirt—and tighten pores. Toners and refreshers that *don't* contain alcohol are usually best suited for men over 40. A mild toner can be effective between washings for removing grime. Apply these with a cotton ball, not a tissue.

Exfoliation

Exfoliation occurs when dead skin cells rise to the surface of the skin's outer layer and are "sloughed off" through washing, shedding, or other means. It is an important process not just for reasons of cleanliness or usefulness to the skin but also because dead cells on the skin's surface tend to dull the skin's appearance. Natural exfoliation can be helped along daily by the use of such abrasives as mild scrubs or oatmeal-based soaps. Once-a-week exfoliant scrubs are becoming increasingly popular for men, and masks (which are designed according to skin types) applied once a week perform the same job. If you are like most men, shaving is probably the best way to exfoliate your way to a healthy sheen.

A "good" shave is of crucial importance to maintaining the skin's health. When men talk about getting a "bad" shave, their most frequent complaints concern cuts and an inability to achieve optimum "closeness"; but improper shaving can also result in flaky or overly dry skin. Using the proper shaving cream (preferably one of the gels that are now readily available) and moisturizing afterward with a cream-based (not an alcohol-based) aftershave should effectively counter such a condition. Luckily, most of today's shaving-cream and aftershave manufacturers have realized that if they want to stay in business they must include more lubricating and moisturizing elements in their products. However, adding a moisturizer to your shaving routine will ensure that your face receives the protection it deserves.

Moisturizers

Moisturizing is the other vital ingredient in the post-40 man's skin-care regimen; and it is especially important now given the skin's increasing tendency at this age to be dry and flaky. Although moisturizers do not replace lost oils or moisture, most act as either a "barrier" to moisture loss or as an "attractor" of moisture from the environment. The *barrier* variety, such as petroleum jelly or those lotions containing lanolin (a greasy wax processed from wool), form a film on the skin that slows the evaporation process. (These usually perform best for the older man.) The latter, *humectant* moisturizers, contain ingredients such as allantoin, urea, elastin, and collagen that have a natural affinity for water and so "bind" environmental moisture to the skin, thus creating a moisturizing effect.

Keep in mind that moisturizing such trouble spots as the chest, shoulders, and back, where perspiration and bacteria tend to build up, is also important. As most women already know, skin care should be directed at the entire body—not just the hands and face.

Beyond these fundamentals there are a few other aspects of skin care that men should be aware of. Some of them—most notably plastic surgery—have heretofore been sought out primarily by women. But the skin-care revolution has led most men to do something of an about-face regarding their personal habits, and they are making full use of the techniques and options available to them.

Let's Review

Here's how you should clean and protect your face:

- First, gently wash with a soap product designed for your skin type. Rinse well with lukewarm water.
- Then, with a cotton ball apply astringent (oily skin), refresher (normal to dry skin), or a toner (sensitive skin).
- Next, exfoliate with a gentle facial scrub (for normal or oily skin use only once or twice a week). First apply hot water to open pores, then lightly massage scrub in a circular motion. Rinse well with warm water.
- Finally, apply moisturizer to your damp skin. If your skin is oily, use a moisturizer labeled non-comeodegenic. It won't clog pores.

Age Spots and Actinic Keratoses

According to the National Institute on Aging, many age-related skin changes, as well as most skin cancers, are surgically correctable. Age spots, also called liver spots, are dark patches usually caused by prolonged exposure to the sun. They occur most often on the backs of hands, but they can also be found on the chest, back, and face. They can be treated with over-the-counter preparations containing hydroquinone, which will lighten the spots. For a more extensive treatment, a doctor can prescribe some relatively simple procedures such as stronger bleaching agents, acid, cryotherapy (a freezing technique using liquid nitrogen), or a curette (scraping) to remove the spots altogether.

Keratoses are sun-induced cancerous lesions on the skin. Actinic keratoses are premalignant in that they only become malignant—and therefore threatening—if left untreated. They are more unsightly than age spots, being greasy, scaly, and brown. A doctor removes them with a scalpel, a curette, or an electric needle through cryotherapy. Repeated applications of a chemical called trichloroacetic acid are also effective at removing the spots.

The sun is also the prime culprit in the most common of all cancers—basal cell carcinoma, which afflicts some 400,000

Americans every year. It is an age-related condition only in that a longer lifetime affords more of a chance for prolonged exposure to the sun. Actually, says the Skin Cancer Foundation, the average age of onset of the disease has steadily decreased. The good news is that skin cancer is also the most curable form of cancer—fully 90 percent of all cases can be cured if they are caught in time.

With early detection so important, you should pay special attention to the state of any sores, moles, rashes, or other growths on your skin. If these change their color, size, shape, and thickness, continue to itch, bleed, crust, or scab, or resist healing, you should have them checked out by a doctor or skin specialist at once. (These symptoms also apply to the other two main types of skin cancer: squamous cell carcinoma and malignant melanoma.)

The physician or dermatologist will perform a biopsy to determine whether the growth is benign, precancerous, or cancerous. Treatment is usually some form of surgery: electrosurgery (the most popular method, in which electricity is used to "burn" away the problem skin); mohs surgery—the method with the highest cure rate (in which excision of the growth is microscopically monitored so that a large amount of healthy tissue can be left intact); excisional surgery (removing the growth); cryosurgery; radiation therapy; and laser surgery. Reconstructive surgery is often needed after these procedures to fully restore the skin's normal appearance.

The best way to avoid having to go through any of this is, simply, to use sunscreens with SPFs of fifteen or more and to avoid prolonged exposure to the sun.

Sunscreens

The sun's ultraviolet rays do more damage to the collagen and support system of skin than anything else. Besides hastening the aging process by causing wrinkles and brown spots, the National Institute of Aging reports that an estimated 300,000 cases of skin cancer occur each year as a result of overexposure to the sun. As we've seen, if detected early, these are usually easily cured. But these statistics alone contradict the popular notion that a tanned body is the epitome of healthy-looking skin. In fact, tanning is only the body's defense mechanism against even more serious damage (though damage may occur even if burning is not evident to the naked eye). Ultraviolet rays chemically change the skin, making it tougher, more leathery, and more wrinkled.

Men of all ages should use sunscreens—at all times—if they are to avoid a sun-induced quickening of the aging process. The most effective of these contain a vitamin known as PABA (para-amino-benzoic acid) and benzophenone derivatives and absorb damaging ultraviolet rays. Other sunscreens use other chemicals to block out the sun's rays. Most sunscreens now on the market are manufactured to meet a system of standards developed by the FDA known as the Sun Protection Factor (SPF), in which consumers are given a choice of how much protection to use (2 to 25). Dermatologists recommend using those with SPF ratings of 15 and above.

Sunscreens should be worn every day—ultraviolet rays do penetrate clouds. Just because it's not sunny out doesn't mean you're safe from the sun! Many moisturizing products now contain sunscreen, so check the label to see if you're getting any protection from your moisturizer. Of course, you should cover *any* part of your skin exposed to the sun's rays, but the bald or balding man should pay particular attention to his pate. Since sunscreens can "goop up" any hair you have left, you might consider wearing a hat whenever you're out of doors.

Dermabrasion and Chemical Peels

These are methods of restoring a youthful appearance by removing fine lines on the surface of skin that has been scarred by acne, blemishes, rashes, or other processes—including aging. Each is becoming more common and can be performed in a doctor's office or in a hospital. They are considered drastic and expensive measures that may be appropriate in only a limited number of cases. Dermabrasion—a controversial procedure—involves "planing" the skin with a wire wheel, a wire brush, or laser beams to strip away the top layers of skin. Performed under a local anesthetic, dermabrasion takes about half an hour.

A chemical peel does the same thing by using a chemical solution to "burn" away the old skin, causing a new layer of smoother skin to form underneath it. Both of these procedures are safe but can take as long as three months to recover from and entail avoiding sunlight for several months thereafter, while the "new" skin grows in. The risks involve loss of pigment (particularly in men with darker complexions) and a variety of irritating circumstances during the healing process.

Collagen Injections

Approved by the Food and Drug Administration several years ago, collagen injections are considered a helpful and safe innovation for use in "plumping up" depressed areas of facial skin. The artificial liquid collagen, derived from animal hides and processed so that it is virtually identical to human collagen, is injected into the wrinkles on your face. Its effects aren't permanent, however. The injections usually wear off after six months to two years, leading many people to get periodic follow-up shots.

Plastic Surgery

Plastic surgery is said by some to be the "ultimate" de-aging process and by others to be a vain, unnatural, and costly attempt (usually not covered by medical insurance) to forestall the inevitable. Surgeons report that in the last few years face-lifts, neck-lifts, eyelid surgery, nose reshaping, and ear reduction are being sought out by increasing numbers of men. There is no denying that in some cases plastic surgery can vastly improve a man's appearance and instill in him newfound confidence. Keep in mind, however, that the effects of many procedures wear off after about five or ten years.

A physician or specialist will be able to give you realistic advice as to what plastic surgery might do for you. Be sure that any surgeon you choose is a member of the AMA and the American College of Surgeons and is on the staff of a major accredited hospital. You can expect to pay between $3,000 and $6,000 for a face-lift.

Nutrition for Healthy Skin

Following a well-balanced diet is as important to one's skin as it is to every other aspect of personal health. Be especially wary of fad weight-loss programs in general but particularly those that limit your intake of fluids. Water is one of the skin's best friends, and lack of moisture in your body's tissues makes itself most evident in the skin.

Alcohol dehydrates the skin. It also acts as a "vasoconstrictor"—constricting the blood vessels, which in turn restricts the flow of oxygen and nutrients through the blood, ultimately harming the skin. Cigarette smoking also decreases the supply of oxygen to the skin, slowing the circulation of blood to your skin. (Many experts claim to be able to recognize heavy smokers by the distinctly "green" cast of their faces.)

The following are some vitamins that appear to be particularly good for the skin:

- **Vitamin A** helps to replenish skin cells. **Good sources:** milk and other dairy products, eggs, and yellow, orange, and dark green fruits and vegetables.
- **Vitamin B** helps prevent scaling and cracking. **Good sources:** grains, dairy products, eggs, dried beans and peas, legumes, lean meats, poultry, fish, and dark-green vegetables.
- **Vitamin C** is necessary for the manufacture of collagen. **Good sources:** citrus fruits, tomatoes, dark-green vegetables, melons, cabbage, and sweet potatoes.

- **Vitamin E** aids in healing. **Good sources:** vegetable oil and shortening, whole-grain products, liver, leafy green vegetables.

(See Chapter Two for a more comprehensive discussion of nutrition.)

Exercise—For the Face and Body

Opinion is divided regarding the value of facial exercises. Some (including exercise booster Jane Fonda) say the rigors of the facial massage itself are such that they couldn't help having a negative effect on the skin's elasticity, especially at a time when a man's skin is already showing signs of declining flexibility. Others say facial exercises couldn't possibly do any harm and since they stimulate the skin and make you feel more vibrant, prescribe them for these reasons alone.

Facial Exercises

If you do decide to ignore Jane Fonda and give your facial and neck muscles a little bit of a workout, here are a few exercises to try:

- Stick your tongue out as far as you can and hold for a few seconds. Repeat 5 times.
- Open your mouth wide and fling your head back. Then open and close your mouth 10 times.
- Open your mouth very wide and hold it open for 5 seconds. Repeat 5 times.
- Open your eyes wide and hold for 5 seconds. Repeat 5 times.

The virtues of overall bodily exercise are much clearer: improved blood flow and circulation in general, as well as increased metabolism—which doctors say may make it possible to speed up the nourishment of skin cells. Adequate rest and sleep—which will no doubt be byproducts of strenuous exercise—are also beneficial in promoting younger-looking skin. Bags and circles under the eyes after late nights age any face. And since exercise and sleep also reduce stress—a common cause of rashes, pimples, and "tired-looking" skin, there's little doubt that regular exercise is one of the most effective ways to achieve youthful-looking skin.

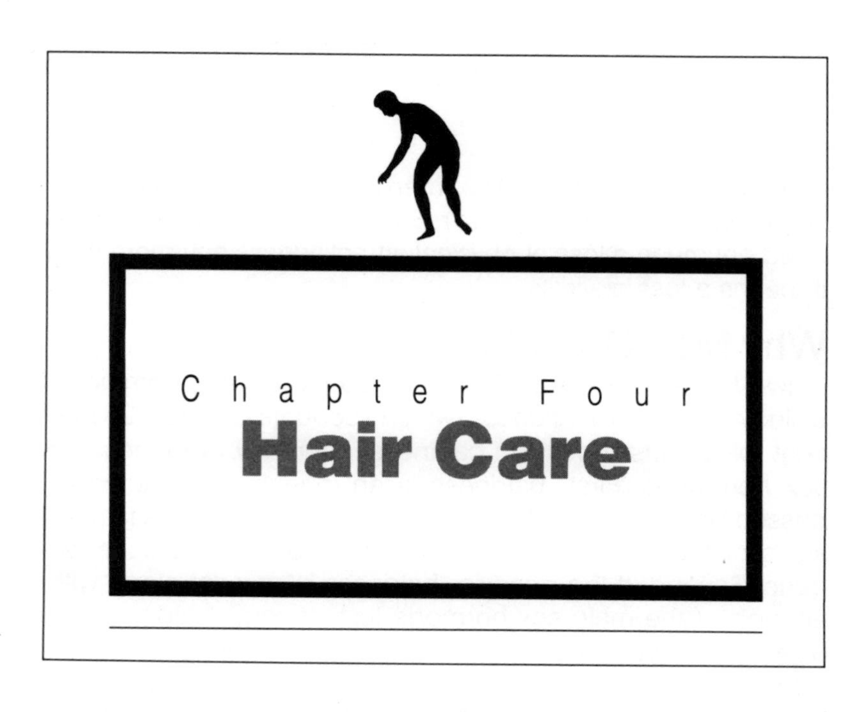

Chapter Four
Hair Care

History is rife with tales of hairy heroes—Samson is probably the most famous—whose feats of derring-do have popularized the idea that having a great shock of hair confers upon an individual commanding powers of wisdom, authority, and sexiness. While there may or may not be something to this notion, its other main implication—that the opposite is true, or that baldness is tantamount to impotence—is obviously false. Luckily, there is no shortage of proof that baldness can mean greatness—witness the achievements and unmistakable charisma of Aristotle, Shakespeare, and Charles de Gaulle, all of whom were very, very bald.

Nonetheless, while few men seem to worry about graying hair most men persist in thinking that going bald means losing stature, energy, and virility—this despite the fact that baldness is a very common state of affairs. According to the *AMA Book of Skin and Hair Care,* baldness occurs in approximately 12 percent of men aged 25, 37 percent of men aged 35, 45 percent of men aged 45, and 65 percent of men aged 65. Other surveys have shown that four out of five men in their 50s and 60s display some evidence of thinning hair. But the prospect of going bald need not mean a loss of physical attractiveness any more than it means a loss of virility.

Why Men Go Bald

Two factors work in tandem to produce what is commonly called *male pattern baldness* (which accounts for about 95 percent of all instances of baldness): heredity, and the male sex hormones. First, baldness is an inherited characteristic passed down in equal parts from the mother's and the father's sides of the families and is transmitted by a sex-influenced gene. Second, if the gene for baldness is present along with enough of the male sex hormone testosterone, baldness will develop. Ironically, testosterone is one of the androgens that, at puberty, helps stimulate the emergence of several male sex traits, among them the growth of body hair, muscle development, deepening of the voice, and development of the sex drive. (Thus males castrated before puberty—when the production of testosterone begins—never become bald.) Even more ironically, the presence of the female hormone estrogen has been found to promote healthy hair and has been shown to be capable of stopping or reversing the genetically mandated balding process. However, one of the several clearly undesirable side effects of this kind of treatment is a diminished sex drive.

What Can and Cannot Be Done About Baldness

Every era has its "snake oil" salesmen. Today's incarnation is the person who claims that through the simple use of his (pick one) lotion, potion, or special formula a man can achieve a miraculous rejuvenation of hair growth that will have him feeling (pick one or more) younger, handsome, more sexually charged. Pay no attention to such characters—an FDA spokesman recently said their claims and gimmicks were all worthless. In fact, the FDA has acted to ban all such products and to require the manufacturers of any future "solutions" to prove their product's effectiveness before it can be sold.

Baldness is first noticed as a V-shaped recession of the hairline and/or the development of a bald patch at the back of the head. If both occur, they will most likely meet and become one at some point. But one of the peculiar aspects of balding is that it does not happen uniformly over time; in other words, a bald area may not change its size for many years. Still, this does not alter the fact that the balding process already has gotten well under way—a fact that is not lost on the many men seeking some way out of their "predicament."

There is is one proven recourse for bald men who want to recoup some of their loss: a hair transplant. Recent estimates place the number of transplants performed by dermatologists and plastic surgeons at about 10,000 per year and on the rise.

The "punch graft" technique devised by noted dermatologist Norman Orentreich in the late 1950s is now considered a mainstream procedure and is the most effective. The only requirement is that the man seeking a punch graft have a suitable amount of "donor" hair. The process involves removing small tufts of hair (including the hair follicles) from areas where the hair is still growing—usually the back and sides of the head—and grafting them (about 20 tufts per session)—to where the hair is desired. A transplant usually requires grafting about 200 to 300 tufts; the operation can be performed once or twice a week.

A number of other techniques—hair weaving, scalp flaps, and scalp-reduction surgery—use different and usually more complex methods to achieve the same results. The procedures vary in cost, effectiveness, durability, and the amount of pain one must endure. You should consult a doctor for help in weigh-

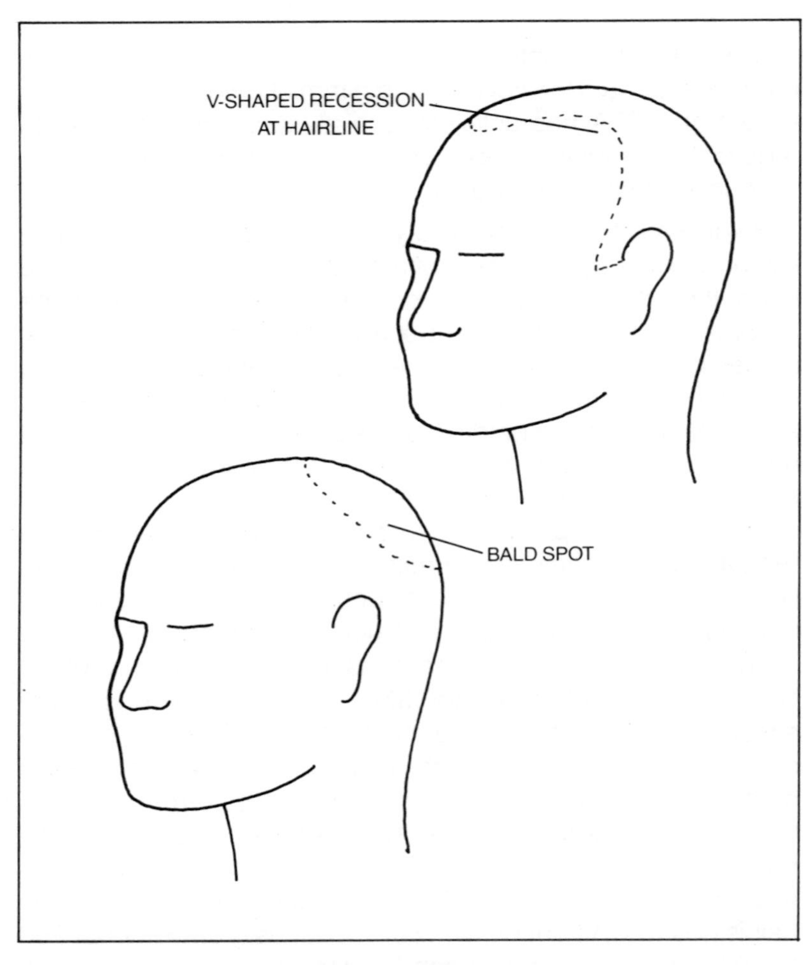

Male Pattern Baldness

ing the relative merits of each.

And since there is still room for improvement in the field, research goes on—one experiment currently under way seeks to perfect the cloning of the part of the hair follicle that is responsible for hair growth, thus creating two half-follicles each capable of growing a full-sized hair. There have been some limited but promising results with topical application of a drug known as minoxidil, which is normally used to combat high blood pressure but whose potential as a baldness treatment came to light when hypertensive patients being given the drug began to show an inordinate amount of hair growth. (One doctor jokes that the patients had begun to look like werewolves.) Early indications are that the drug—applied topically in lotion form—may be more effective as a way to *stave off* or *delay* baldness—and even then only in very limited cases—than as a way to generate large amounts of new growth for already-bald individuals. One doctor told *Esquire* magazine that "the best you can expect at this point is that minoxidil will bring you back to where you were five years earlier—the shorter the length of time you have been losing hair and the smaller the loss, the better the results."

Minoxidil has been approved by the FDA, but only as a treatment for hypertensives. The organization is now closely reviewing its use as a baldness curative and is said to be concerned about its potency. As one doctor told *People* magazine, "They don't want it being absorbed through the skin and causing blood pressures to drop and people to faint all over the place." So far, however, no significant side effects have been reported, and it is becoming more widely available (a pharmacist must convert it to the lotion form).

Bald and Proud of It

Of course, you might be the sort of person who prefers not to seek any of these "remedies." Allowing nature to take its course is a perfectly reasonable choice, particularly if surgery doesn't appeal to you. But more importantly because it is a realistic—and confidence-building—approach to a perfectly natural life change. You're not about to don a toupee—which almost always looks fake no matter how expensive—nor do you want to let what hair you have grow so long that you can use it to cover your bald spots (a widespread practice). That just looks awkward.

One of the more sensible things you can do is to cultivate your facial hair—beards and moustaches are attractive ways to focus attention on your face and to help you regain some of whatever virility you feel you might have lost. But most of all, don't worry about it. Baldness can be sexy—particularly if you *feel* sexy.

The Advantages of Graying

Gray hair is something many men seem to enjoy and many women find extremely attractive on men. It is another normal part of the aging process, but *when* you start to turn gray depends upon heredity. Most men in their middle 40s already show some gray and find that its connotations of aging are tempered by the aura of dignity and sophistication that many people ascribe to the gray-haired man. The softer tones of gray hair also have a brightening effect on a man's older face, enlivening his general appearance. And gray hair is often thicker, filling out thinning hair.

Because of its genetic and age-related causes, graying is not reversible except through hair coloring. The majority of men prefer to leave their hair gray; but if you're uncomfortable with the color of your hair, don't worry about changing it. A professional will advise you on the best treatments to match your natural color. At-home treatments—those you wash into your hair—tend to look unnatural. (*Warning:* Hair dyes made of coal-tar derivatives have caused cancer in lab rats and mice. Avoid products containing the ingredient 4MMOD.)

Hair Care

The important thing is to keep the hair you do have looking healthy. The following hair-care tips should be made part of your routine:

- Most men should shampoo and condition daily, unless you find your hair becoming overly dry or oily. End your shampoo with a cold-water rinse; it heightens shine.
- Be sure to select shampoos based on your hair type, and make sure you don't feel any "stripping" or abrasion while lathering up—this could be a sign that the shampoo is too harsh for your hair.
- Don't overuse your blow dryer; letting your hair dry naturally or using the blow dryer when it's partially dry helps it retain more of a glow.
- Be gentle while brushing your hair, and never brush wet hair (use a wide-toothed comb).
- Get your hair cut every four to six weeks to give it a fuller, thicker look.
- Treat dandruff promptly. Dandruff shampoos do help. Keep in mind, too, that dandruff can also occur if you don't rinse your hair properly after shampooing—soap and shampoo particles remain on the scalp and dry it out. There is also some evidence that not eating a well-balanced diet can cause dandruff.
- Don't forget to shampoo your moustache and beard daily and condition them once a week. Blow-drying will make the beard softer but may also dry out your skin.

Nutrition

Nutrition is also an important part of your daily hair care. A well-balanced diet—rich in vitamins—should keep your hair looking and feeling healthy. But if it doesn't, consider the following:

- **Calories.** If your diet doesn't include enough calories, your hair shows it. A starvation diet starves your hair as well as your body.

- **Amino acids.** These are the building blocks of protein and are essential for healthy hair. **Good sources:** meat, milk, cheese, and eggs. (Strict vegetarians may have a problem with their hair.)
- **Vitamin F.** Another name for fatty acids, which lubricate and condition the hair follicles. In a normal diet the oils used in cooking and the fat in meat are generally all you'll need.
- **Iron.** Anemia may cause hair to become dull and brittle, and it is a common cause of hair loss, so it's important to be sure you get enough iron. **Good sources:** meat, organ meats, poultry, egg yolks, and dried beans.
- **B-Complex Vitamins.** If you don't get enough, your scalp may become scaly and red, and your hair may lose its color and shine. **Good sources:** dried beans and peas, dairy products, eggs, lean meats, poultry, organ meats, fish, and dark-green vegetables.
- **Vitamin C.** This vitamin helps to keep your capillaries healthy so that they can carry blood to your hair follicles. **Good sources:** citrus fruits, strawberries, cabbage, dark-green vegetables, melons, tomatoes, and sweet potatoes.

(See Chapter 2 for more about good nutrition.)

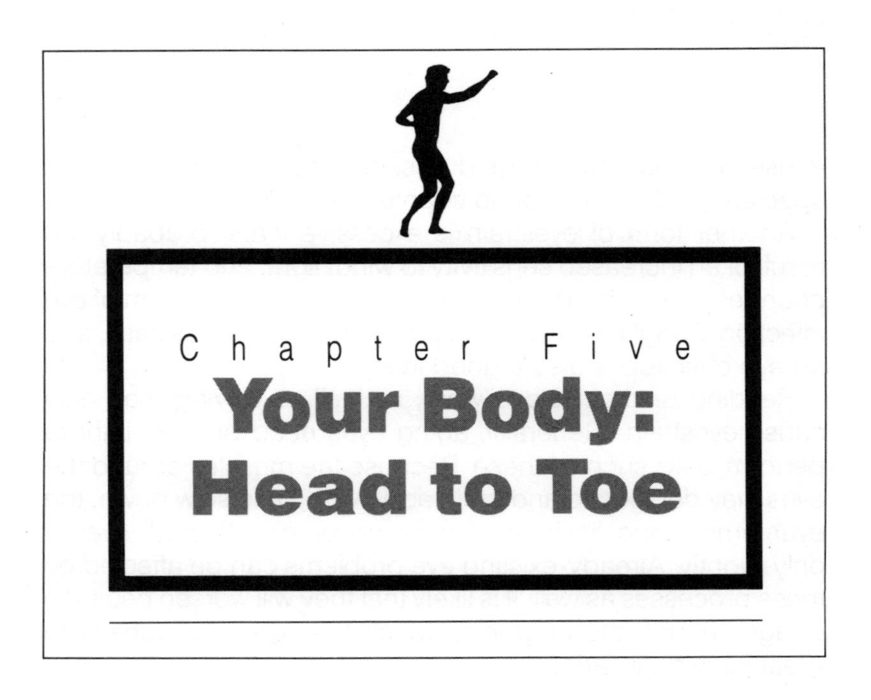

Chapter Five
Your Body: Head to Toe

There are a lot of bodily changes that occur with age. Some can cause medical problems. Many of them are not serious—merely annoying—and many of the changes associated with aging can be easily and effectively controlled—through exercise, proper nutrition, and in some cases, medical treatment. This chapter covers some of those changes.

For Your Eyes Only

Though poor eyesight is not an inevitable result of aging, a man in his 40s or 50s may experience a variety of physical changes that can affect his vision. However, although this period of a man's life has often been called the "bifocal age," a man can in fact maintain good eyesight well into his advanced years.

Certain age-related changes in the eye's support system can cause eye strain, and one common manifestation of eye strain is dry eyes, which result because aging tear glands may produce too few tears with which to irrigate the eyes. Symptoms are itching, burning, and even reduced vision. You may decide to use over-the-counter eye drops, but doctors can prescribe a special eye-drop solution to counter the problem.

Another form of eyestrain is excessive tears, probably the result of an increased sensitivity to wind, light, and temperature changes, but a condition that may also signal some form of eye infection. Sunglasses can help protect the eyes in this case, and an eye checkup is also a good idea.

Reading or other close work, as well as driving, can also cause eyestrain. Generally, aging eyes need brighter light to perform tasks such as these. Because the muscles around the eyes may deteriorate and brain activity begin to slow down, the eye's timing and flexibility can be adversely affected, even if only slightly. Already-existing eye problems can be affected by these processes as well. It is likely that they will worsen because of age, though the degree to which they do so is subject to great individual variation.

Presbyopia

One of the most common age-related eye problems faced by men in their middle years is presbyopia, a condition that causes farsightedness and occurs because the eye's crystalline lens begins to lose its ability to change its shape and is less able to focus nearby objects on the retina. To counteract this vision problem, many men opt for bifocals, in which the upper lens is geared for seeing distances and the lower lens is designed for reading or other close work.

Cataracts

Less common but not unknown among men of this age are cataracts, which are areas of the lens that become opaque and shut out light, thus impairing vision. There are a variety of theories regarding the reason cataracts develop. Some say that cataracts will occur in anyone who lives long enough—the implication being that it is a natural reaction to the wear and tear life places on one's vision. One ophthalmologist, however, citing his experience with nutritionally deficient Ethiopians who developed cataracts as early as their 30s and 40s, says that the underlying cause is dietary. Still others cite the ability of free radicals to initiate oxidation and tissue alteration in the lens.

Cataracts can be surgically removed if they have grown large enough to interfere with vision (some remain small and cause no harm). The procedure is safe and nearly always successful. Special glasses or lens implants are then required to restore one's eyesight. Doctors have also found that vitamin and mineral supplements of zinc, vitamin A, vitamin B, and vitamin B_2 (riboflavin) are effective both as preventive measures and in reversing the formation of cataracts.

Glaucoma

Glaucoma, in which an imbalance of eye fluid creates abnormally high fluid pressure in the eye, which in turn causes internal eye damage, is one of the leading causes of blindness for men over the age of 35. It is particularly bedeviling because it affects so many people—an estimated 1,000,000 people in the United States suffer from glaucoma—while having no known cause. Early diagnosis and treatment usually can control or prevent serious glaucoma damage. Often, however, irreparable damage is done before the condition is diagnosed, since any symptoms are rarely exhibited. Treatment consists of special eye drops, oral medications, laser treatments, and, in some cases, surgery.

Among the many things a man can do to protect himself from all types of eye problems are the following:

- Maintain proper nutritional habits, including vitamin supplements. Vitamin A, which has been shown to improve night vision, can be found in carrots, squash, spinach, fortified milk, liver, and eggs. Vitamin C—low levels of which have been linked to cataracts and glaucoma—can be found in dark-green vegetables, citrus fruits, and

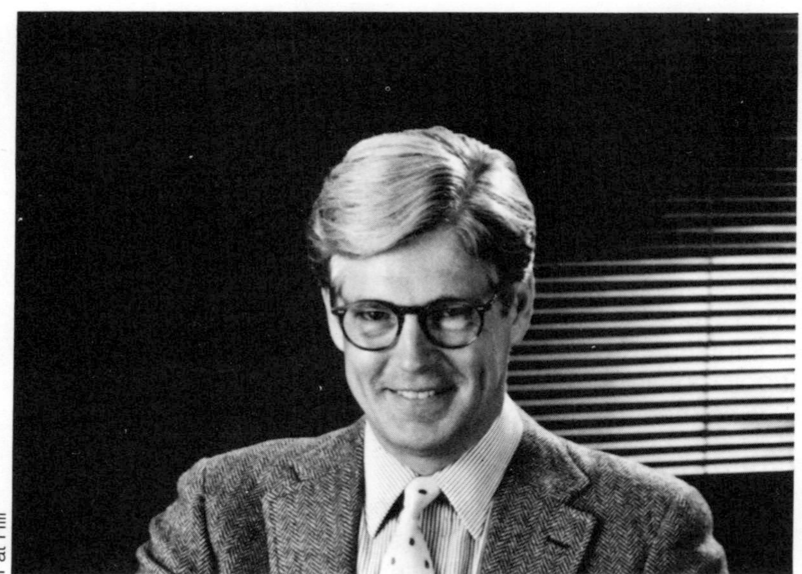

Pat Hill

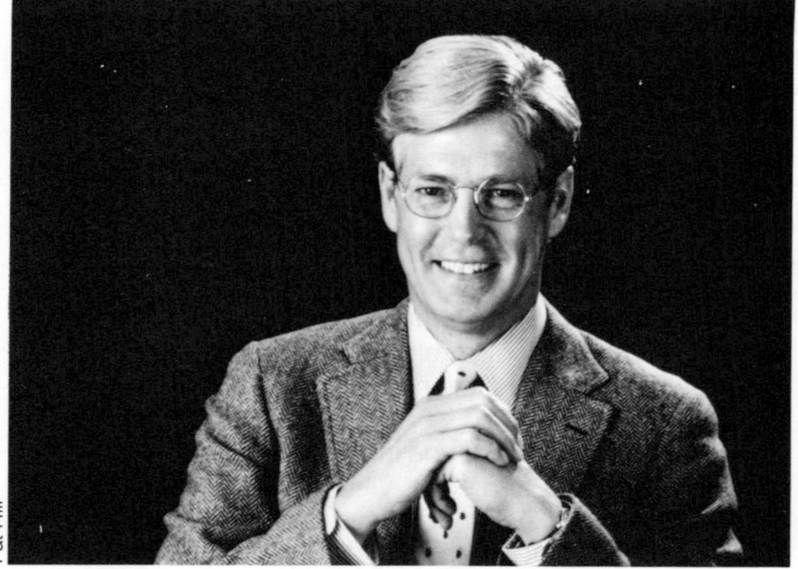

Pat Hill

tomatoes.

- Wear protective glasses during athletic activity or during work in which debris may fill the air.
- Wear sunglasses—the lenses should be green or brown —when appropriate. (Don't wear them all the time, however; the adjustment of your eyes to various degrees of light and dark is good for them.)
- Always have adequate light with which to read or work. This prevents eyestrain.
- Get a sufficient amount of sleep—your eyes need time to relax.
- Perform these simple eye exercises: Closing them purposely during the day for brief periods of time gives them a chance to relax; blinking lubricates and cleanses them. Focusing exercises, a sort of target practice for the eyes, are espoused by behavioral optometrists as a way to condition the eyes to see better by strengthening muscles.
- Get an eye examination every two years.
- If you already wear glasses, have your prescription checked regularly.
- Don't use eye drops more than once a day.
- Don't stare at a computer screen for more than an hour without taking a 5-minute break.

Eye Wear

As the treatment of eye disease has become more sophisticated, so has eye wear itself. For those of you who can't stand the frequent attention that must be paid to contact lenses, the development of "extended wear" contact lenses—which can be worn for as long as a week without being removed—is rendering that complaint obsolete. Especially promising for the man in the "bifocal age" has been the creation of bifocal contact lenses, which are slightly more expensive but are probably a bargain considering their convenience.

And finally, for those of you who perceive glasses as one of life's cumbersome and unattractive necessities, remember—the ever-increasing variety of styles available means that glasses have attained a heightened status as a fashion element and a mode of self-expression. Better style—and better sight—can be yours for as long as you live.

Healthy Hearing

Hearing loss is another sign of aging. You begin by having a little trouble hearing high-frequency sounds. A man usually begins to lose his capacity for hearing at age 50, a decline that continues at a very gradual pace. By age 65, however, the condition might be considerably more pronounced. According to the National Institute on Aging, about 30 percent of adults age 65 through 74, and half of those age 75 through 79, exhibit some degree of hearing loss.

Most ear experts—called otologists and audiologists—point to aging and the rigors of everyday life in noisy Western society as the prime culprits for hearing loss. Some indication as to the power of the effects of environment was given by the results of a study that tested the hearing ability of members of a primitive tribe living in isolation in Africa. Most of them—no matter what age—were able to hear a whisper from as far away as 100 yards!

Deafness

Hearing disabilities come in two varieties. The first is *conduction deafness,* in which the ear's ability to conduct sound impulses is impaired by a buildup of ear wax or some other substance, a blockage of the eustachian tube in the inner ear (most commonly caused by an infection), or a punctured eardrum. *Nerve deafness,* on the other hand, means that the actual nerve fibers, cells, and other elements of the inner ear have somehow been damaged—most likely by the existence of excess inner-ear fluid, the effects of excess noise over time, or through simple wear and tear. The most common form of nerve deafness is known as *presbycusis.* Nerve deafness may cause dizzy spells, since the body's balance mechanism, located in the inner ear, may be affected.

Unfortunately, aside from keeping your ears clean and free of wax (with a cotton swab; be careful not to penetrate too deeply), avoiding excessive noise when possible, covering your ears in winter, and having your hearing tested every few years, there is not much that can be done to prevent hearing loss. Treatment of hearing difficulties may involve the simple flushing out of excess ear wax (easily done in a doctor's office), surgery, or other measures. A doctor's advice should be sought if your hearing loss is so advanced that a hearing aid might be necessary. Even if you have no apparent hearing trouble, a periodic visit to the ear doctor—once a year after age 55—is recommended.

Your Teeth

First, the good news: As you get older you will probably get fewer cavities—maybe even none. Now the bad news: The odds are high that you will get some form of periodontal disease—which accounts for about 75 percent of all tooth loss in people over 40. The American Dental Association estimates that over half of all adults over age 18 have some form of periodontal disease and more specifically that two out of every three middle-aged men in America show some signs of tooth-threatening gum disease.

Thus, the oral-hygiene program for a man over 40 places increasing emphasis on the gums—although you still must pay attention to the prevention of cavities. *Remember:* It is not aging but bacteria that cause tooth decay. Aging simply creates more opportunities and time for bacteria to do their damage and more time for the effects of poor tooth-care habits to add up. Tooth experts—the American Dental Association among them—believe that many people over the age of 40 approach tooth care from a defeatist perspective: that tooth loss is an inevitable part of aging. Such an attitude is particularly damaging at an age when certain aspects of tooth and gum care become most critical.

Periodontal Disease

Periodontal disease is particularly insidious because by the time it becomes noticeable it has, most likely, already done substantial harm to the gums. It is caused by the buildup of bacterial plaque and its byproducts, which harden into calculus (also known as tartar)—which in turn makes removing any new plaque more problematic. As the gums become increasingly irritated, they pull away from the teeth, leaving small pockets into which more plaque may move, ultimately enlarging the pockets and finally—in the most severe cases—attacking and destroying the tissue and bone that support the teeth. By this advanced stage the teeth may become loose, may fall out altogether, or may be so far beyond repair that a dentist has no choice but to remove them. In this day and age, however, there is little excuse for allowing periodontal disease to progress so far.

Early detection of periodontal disease is crucial. The ADA suggests a visit to the dentist if you show any of the following symptoms:

1. gums that bleed when you brush your teeth
2. gums that are red, swollen, or tender
3. gums that have pulled away from the teeth
4. pus between the teeth and gums when the gums are pressed
5. permanent teeth that are loose or separating
6. any change in the way your teeth fit together when you bite
7. any changes in the fit of your partial dentures
8. bad breath

You can help lessen the likelihood that periodontal disease

will be a problem for you if you:

- Brush twice daily with a fluoride toothpaste, using a small brush with soft, end-rounded bristles.
- Replace brushes every three or four months.
- Floss thoroughly (for several minutes) once a day. It's the only way to get rid of plaque. (Extra-fine unwaxed floss is the best kind.)
- Brush your tongue every time you brush. (The tongue is another nesting ground for bacteria.)
- Eat a balanced diet, with an absolute minimum of sweets and processed foods containing sugar. Without the proper nutrients, periodontal disease progresses faster and heals more slowly.
- Remember that electric toothbrushes are no better than manual ones and that water sprays don't substitute for flossing. Neither is harmful, however.
- Visit your dentist regularly, some say as often as two or three times per year.
- Brush with a paste made of two tablespoons of baking soda and a small amount of hydrogen peroxide: first—using a rubber applicator (the type that comes on the end of some toothbrushes)—massage the paste onto the teeth, paying particular attention to the gum line. Then, brush and rinse. If you are left with an unpleasant taste in your mouth, you can brush again using your regular toothpaste. Some dentists even recommend sleeping with the paste in the mouth, to give the mixture extra time to fight plaque buildup. This procedure can be done every night, but even once or twice a week will prove beneficial.

Cavities

According to the ADA, two out of three caries (cavities) in people over 50 years old are caused by decay that accumulates around fillings. Because men entering their 40s and 50s today are likely to have many fillings—having grown up without the benefits of fluoridated water or fluoride toothpastes—this type of cavity presents a significant problem. Among tooth caries, root canals are particularly prevalent in this age group, mostly because of the gum recession fostered by periodontal disease. The same preventive measures as those used to fight periodontal disease are recommended here.

Reconstructive Dentistry

According to the ADA about one third of the U.S. population twenty years ago wore full dentures. That figure has dropped to less than 20 percent today and is expected to decline even further in coming years. However, these statistics should not inspire complacency about tooth and gum care—as we've seen, the utmost diligence is needed to ensure good dental health for as long as we live. Rather, the figures illustrate the advances that have been made in reconstructive dentistry, which not only has helped more people to retain more of their natural teeth longer than previous generations could have expected, but also has made discolored, cracked, or chipped teeth look as good as new.

For instance, orthodontic care is now being sought by large numbers of adults. Of all patients seeking to straighten their teeth and better their bites through the use of braces, fully 15 percent of them are adults, a percentage that is rising steadily. This can be attributed to an increased public awareness of the importance of a proper bite to good dental health and also to the fact that braces themselves do their job more quickly and have become less unsightly and easier to clean. Some can be worn on the inside (or back) of the teeth, others are made in clear or tooth-colored materials, and still others are held in place by glue, a marked improvement over unattractive metal bands.

Work to repair teeth or improve their appearance with caps, crowns, bridges, and partial and full dentures continues, of course, with ever more sophisticated and realistic-looking materials (and less painful techniques). Probably the most popular method is "bonding," a procedure developed in the 1950s in which the teeth are coated and cured with various acrylic and filling materials that are sculpted to cover areas with particular problems and then lightened to give a bright—but not unrealistic—appearance. The effects are said to last about five to eight years; no anesthesia or drilling is required, but bonding is not as durable as a cap (though it is less expensive). Laminate veneers—which have been compared to false fingernails—have also proven popular as a less-expensive and fairly durable cosmetic technique.

Your dentist and the ADA can apprise you of the latest developments in the field and which procedure may be right for you.

Oh, My Aching Back!

There is nothing about back pain that a man can't cure. That might be news to the estimated 75 million Americans who suffer from back trouble, but it's true. Admittedly, the man who goes through life without experiencing low-back syndrome or disc trouble is considered something of a modern medical marvel.

Back pain is no excuse for abandoning exercise. In fact, it's a reason to start. Stretching exercises, yoga, low-stress aerobics, and swimming—a sport that doesn't place any stress on the spine—all help strengthen your body. In addition, back pain can be eliminated through weight control and paying diligent attention to one's posture.

After age 40 a man's muscle strength begins to decline, a pattern that is related in part to the heart's diminished ability to supply the muscles with blood. Biochemically, the loss of strength occurs because the muscles lose their capacity for storing glycogen (blood glucose converted to a form that can be used by the muscles), which is the fuel used by the muscles when the body is called upon to perform some physical task. At the same time, the spine—that incredibly complex and delicate structure whose main function is the gravity-defying support of our upper bodies—also receives fewer nutrients (including calcium), as the blood supply to the discs diminishes.

Other stresses on the musculoskeletal system normally associated with aging include extra weight around the waist, general abdominal flabbiness, and the accumulated effects of poor posture while standing or sitting. (Some researchers have even speculated that man wasn't meant to stand fully erect, and that had we continued to locomote more as our primate cousins do, back trouble would not occur.) These physical changes occur whether or not a man is healthy, whether or not he is active, whether or not he has kept his muscles limber and in shape through stretching and aerobics. However, the sedentary man is much worse off when these age-related changes begin. This does not mean that such physical changes need to be blindly accepted. There are simple and effective steps that will counteract any pain or discomfort arising from back problems.

Low-Back Syndrome

Whatever the source of the duress, at some point the support system may "give way" under the strain. Low-back syndrome, also known as lumbago—which refers to a region of the lower back called the lumbosacral area at the lower part of the spinal column—is usually set off by a distinct episode of physical overexertion, such as an especially taxing lift or twist. Usually, though, lower-level symptoms of back pain or soreness have been present for quite some time. The pain, usually described as "knifelike" is caused either by an irritation of the spinal nerves or an inflammation of the back muscles. Problems in the spine or in the sciatic nerve (the largest nerve in the body, which is actually two nerves, one each running from the pelvis down the back of the thighs) can also cause pain along the back of the leg and/or thigh.

The severe stabbing pain will usually wear off after a few days, but some symptoms—stiffness, tenderness, lower-level pain—will remain and if not treated will sometimes become chronic (in other words, the discomfort is always felt or easily aggravated by even a mildly strenuous motion, such as a sneeze). The symptoms can be fought with pain-relieving pills, the application of heating pads, and bed rest; but it should be pointed out that such efforts, while helpful, merely attack the symptoms—not the cause.

While many men even acclimate themselves to the constant pain by "taking it easy" or, worse, adjusting their walk, posture, and other body motions so as to avoid triggering pain, this is probably the worst thing you can do. Instead, your best bets are gentle stretching exercises performed carefully and gradually; aerobics, with adequate warming-up and cooling-down periods; weight control through exercise and proper nutrition; and posture practice. Inversion therapy, a recently popular practice in which special boots enable one to hang upside down from a bar—ostensibly straightening and realigning the spine in the process—is a controversial solution. Doctors disagree as to whether inversion therapy works and whether or not it is safe.

You might also consider working at a stand-up desk since sitting all day is the musculoskeletal system's number-one enemy. Or, there are special chairs designed to take the stress off the back. *Note:* Running is not advisable as part of a back-strengthening aerobic regimen because the constant pounding of the body and feet on the ground/track places too much pressure on the spine.

Disc Trouble

Low-back pain may actually be a sign of a "slipped" or herniated disc. The spinal discs—which serve as shock absorbers between the individual vertebrae—consist of a thick outer rim and a pulpy inner mass. When the disc is ruptured—again as a result of some extreme physical exertion or strain—the mass oozes out and puts pressure on a nerve, causing excruciating pain. The pain is so debilitating that immediate bed rest, heating pads, pain relievers, and possibly traction are called for as the first steps toward recovery.

Recently a drug known as *chymopapain,* derived from the papaya plant, has been used widely—as a treatment to relieve pressure on the spinal nerves. Though it was approved by the FDA in 1982 after tests showed a 75 percent success rate, its use is still controversial because some people have displayed an allergic reaction and because it still remains ineffective for a good 25 percent of those who try it. The FDA recommends its use only after treatments such as bed rest and traction fail.

Like other low-back pain, the incidence of slipped discs is at its highest around middle age, owing in part to the age-related changes in the muscles, spine, and bones. Both active and inactive men may be stricken, though the latter are obviously more susceptible because of their weakened muscles and their generally slackened physical condition. Because slipped discs have a tendency to recur, a supervised exercise program geared toward strengthening the back and abdominal muscles is recommended—as are regular exercise and posture awareness once recovery is achieved.

Chiropractic Therapy

Chiropractic therapy is making a comeback. Once dismissed as quackery, the benefits of spinal manipulation have been experienced by some 9½ million Americans (in 1983), among them leading athletes and Olympic competitors whose careers were given new life. While scientific evidence of its effectiveness is still lacking, and the American Medical Association continues to caution against using chiropractors—saying that they too often treat ailments beyond their scope—the empirical evidence suggests that chiropractors can indeed achieve success, often where conventional treatment techniques have failed.

Chiropractors treat everything from backaches to headaches, operating on the theory that if the spine and its associated muscles and nerves are not in proper position and shape the vertebrae will press on nerves, thereby disrupting the flow of "energy" through the body and causing various forms of distress. Through spinal manipulation, massage, exercise therapy, and sound-wave therapy, chiropractors—who are trained and licensed in all fifty states—seek to locate and correct the trouble. Your doctor or the American Chiropractic Association (1916 Wilson Boulevard, Arlington, Virginia 22201) can give you more information if you think a chiropractor could help you.

Arthritis

Perhaps in no other way does the wear and tear of a lifetime so poignantly express itself as in the visible signs of arthritis—stiffness and pain at the joints, making the body creak and snap.

Of the two most common forms of arthritis seen in people over 40—osteoarthritis and rheumatoid arthritis—the former is of greater concern to men. (The latter affects three times as many women as men and is much more debilitating.) By the time they reach their 50s, most men begin to feel the slow, gradually developing signs of osteoarthritis—slight pain in the knees, hips, and spine, the main weight-bearing joints of the body, and perhaps elsewhere as well—all the result of inflamed joints.

Overall, however, the condition is relatively mild. The inflammation is thought to be caused by the usual culprits—general wear and tear, lack of exercise, poor posture, and excess weight, though a full understanding of arthritis has not yet been attained. Severe crippling is rare with this form of arthritis, and countering the suspected causative factors usually results in some improved flexibility and mobility. Although there is no cure for arthritis, several effective treatments are available—aspirin, acetaminophen, non-steroidal anti-inflammatory drugs, and, sometimes, surgery.

Rheumatoid arthritis also baffles health experts and is all the more troubling because of its ability to severely cripple its victims. It appears most frequently in joints such as fingers, wrists, elbows, knees, hips, and ankles, where swelling and spasms increasingly "freeze" the joints, rendering them less and less mobile. What makes rheumatoid arthritis significantly more serious than osteoarthritis is this apparently "infectious" nature of the arthritis process itself. As with osteoarthritis, not much is known about the causes of rheumatoid arthritis; among the suspected factors are stress—both physical and emotional—as well as allergy or some other state of hypersensitivity. Treatment requires taking the same measures as those used to combat osteoarthritis, but obviously the prospects for recovery or lessening pain are not as great.

"Loss of erective prowess is not a natural component of aging." So said William Masters and Virginia Johnson in their famed study of human sexual behavior. They also found that a man should be able to have erections well into his 80s—unless illness or some kind of psychological barrier interferes.

And similar findings have been reported by virtually anyone who looks into the issue, including renowned sex researchers Alfred Kinsey and Shere Hite and the team of Bernard D. Starr and Marcella Bakur Weiner, who wrote in 1981: "Our fear that sexuality—alive and well in our twenties, thirties, and forties—should suddenly atrophy and die as we move into the later decades, makes no more sense than the notion that our ability to enjoy food or smells or conversation will disappear."

Yes, there are distinct changes that occur in the body of the man over 40 that may have some kind of effect on his sex life, but these need not diminish his sexual activity. Quite the contrary. Nonetheless, most men seem to think that when they first sense the perfectly normal "slowing of response" they have reached a depressing, sexually frustrating stage of life. How can a man counteract this tendency and come to acknowledge—as he should—that there are many fulfilling sexual years ahead of him? First and foremost he needs to understand exactly what physiological changes do occur and what they mean.

According to urologist Sherman Silver, author of *The Male,* the aging man (there's no specific age) will experience the following changes:

- The penis will take longer to become erect when aroused.
- It will take a longer period of stimulation to reach orgasm. (This can be something of a blessing for the man who has had difficulty controlling the timing of his ejaculation; or to his partner, who may not have been able to achieve orgasm through intercourse because of the man's swiftness.)
- With each successive year the orgasm will become slightly briefer.
- The force of the ejaculation—and its volume—will diminish with age.
- The penis will most likely return to its flaccid state within moments of orgasm, and a longer period of time will be needed to regain an erect state.

Most changes are the result of a decline in the levels of the body's steroid hormones and are considered normal. However, they can be rather traumatic for the man who is not expecting them or who can't stop recalling his teenage years and thinks his sex life is about to end. Indeed, as Shere Hite reported in *The Hite Report on Male Sexuality,* of all age groups surveyed men 40 to 49 years old expressed the most vehement fears that aging would have a negative effect on their sex lives.

Men should not fear their chronological age: Good health, sufficient exercise, and emotional maturity are the most important components of continued sexual enjoyment. One accurate barometer of what a man can expect for his post-40 sex life is to look at his pre-40 sex life: *Vitality breeds vitality.*

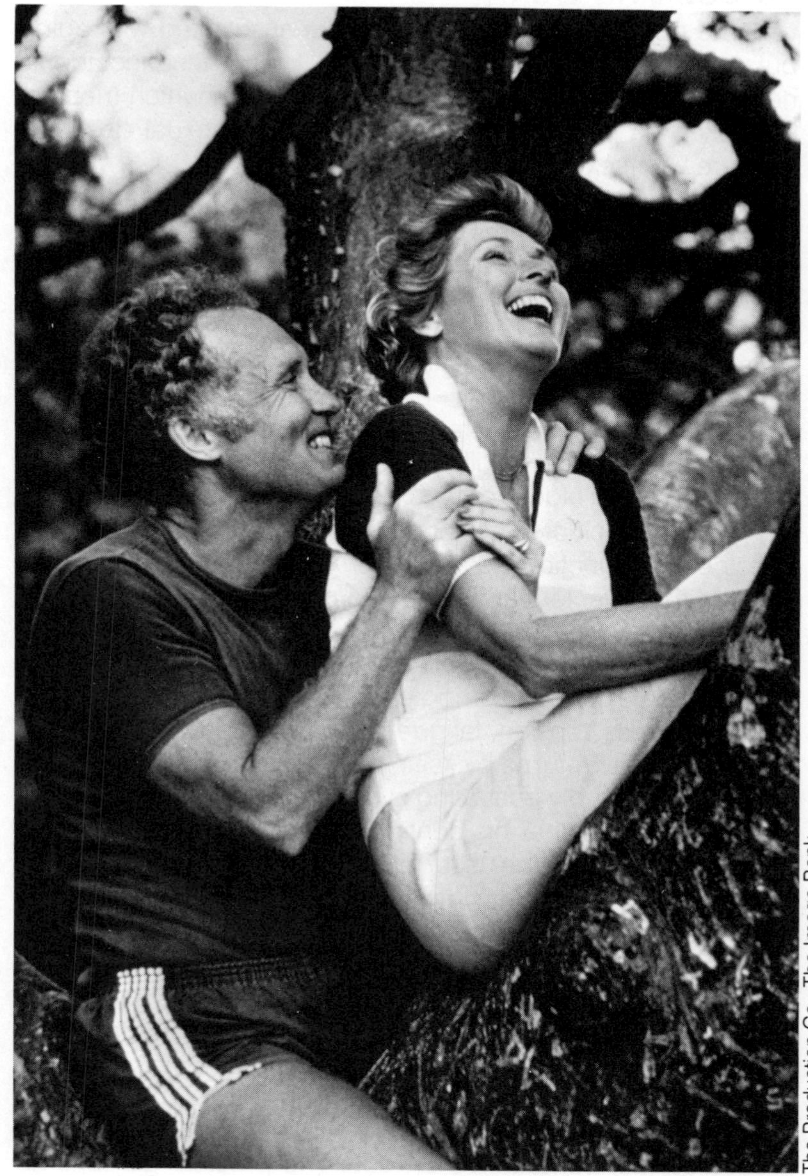

The Production Co., The Image Bank

Illness and Sex

Some physical hindrances to sex are associated with aging but are actually not caused by aging itself. These include illnesses such as diabetes and heart disease, in which medication taken as part of the treatment can dull sexual desire or interfere with sexual capability.

Contrary to the popular notion that having a heart attack means forswearing "stressful" sex, doctors are worried that abstinence may actually cultivate unhealthy tension. According to the National Institute on Aging, sex can usually be resumed within twelve to sixteen weeks; indeed an active sex life—owing to its tranquilizing nature—may have a hand in preventing future attacks.

Drugs taken to relieve stress or tension may also disrupt sexual performance. Other illnesses or chronic ailments take a heavier toll on an older body, sex life included. And, not surprisingly, fatigue, lack of sleep, and overuse of alcohol temporarily impair sexual function—at any age! As we have seen, a good many of these factors are subject to our control.

A Note About Impotence

Most men experience impotence at one time or another because of illness, tension, fatigue, or overindulgence in alcohol. Potency usually returns by itself, but if a man is too worried he may set off a terribly frustrating cycle—fear keeps him impotent at the same time that his continued impotence creates more fear. Fear of failure is the usual feeling reported by younger men going through a bout with impotence. For the man over 40 who is experiencing fear of aging as well as the actual physical manifestations of a slower response, the fears can multiply. It is best to remember that it is the fears and fantasies that are damaging, while the reality—continual sexual fulfillment and satisfaction—can easily be yours with the proper effort and mindset.

The Prostate Gland

Located just beneath the bladder, the prostate gland is an

accessory male reproductive organ whose primary role is to secrete a fluid that stimulates the sperm into greater motility. Without the prostate gland a man is sterile. Probably because of hormonal changes, the gland becomes enlarged in about 10 percent of men over 40, 50 percent of men over 50, and in most men over age 60.

The most common type of prostate trouble is known as benign prostatic hypertrophy. Its symptoms include painful urination, a frequent and urgent need to urinate, pain during erection or orgasm, and other difficulties with urinary excretion—dribbling, slowness of stream, and incomplete emptying of the bladder. If you experience any of these symptoms you should, of course, see a doctor. In some cases a complete blockage of the urinary tract occurs. About 10 percent of men under age 80 require surgery, in which an excess portion of the gland is removed to restore proper urinary function.

Prostatitis, an irregular inflammation of the gland also characterized by a variety of urinary difficulties, can also plague men over 40. In this case, the antibiotic tetracycline is the usual treatment.

Prostate cancer, according to *Jane Brody's The New York Times Guide to Personal Health,* is "the third most common cancer killer of American men and the leading cause of cancer deaths among men aged 70 or beyond." Because its symptoms are, to the patient, just like those of the milder prostate ailments, early detection by a doctor is crucial to prevent further spread of the disease. Accordingly, men over 40 should have an annual rectal exam. Treatment for prostate cancer involves radiation therapy and surgery, with the former thought to have the edge because it does not leave a man impotent.

It has been said that the brain and the skin are the two most powerful sex organs in the body. And, as men enter their 40s they have been shown to realize the importance of emotional intimacy as an integral component of good sex. At the same time, the skin assumes heightened significance as the emphasis on orgasm fades somewhat in favor of a more generalized sense of touch and an awareness of the entire body. In other words, there comes to be much more to a healthy sex life than just having an orgasm. The sooner you realize this, the more gratifying your sex life (and that of your partner) will be.

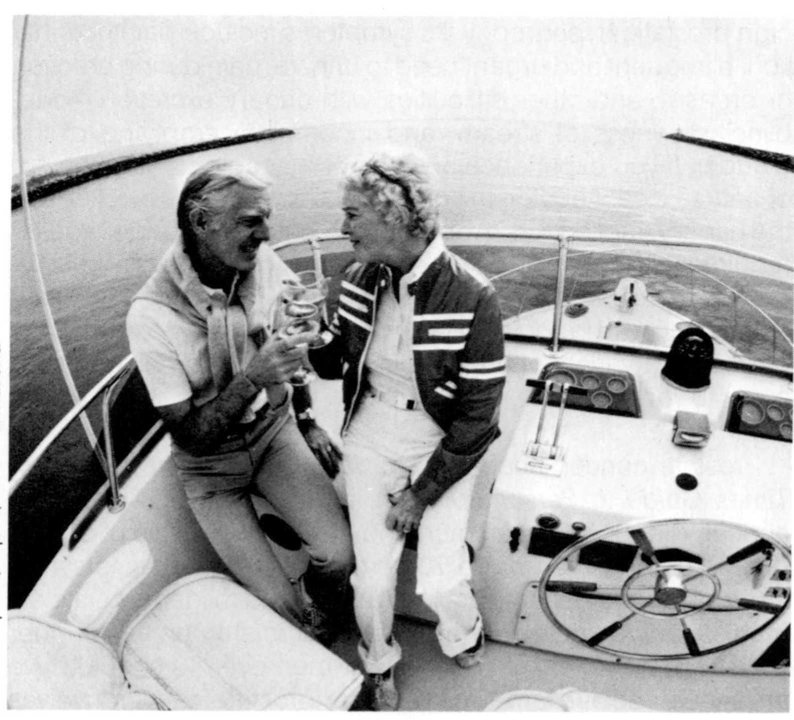

Tom Campbell, Alpha, FPG International

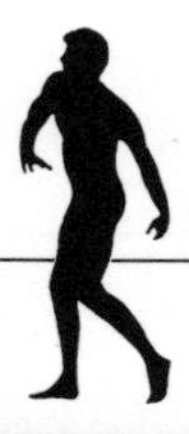

Chapter Seven

Your Mind: Mental and Emotional Health

Coping with Stress

Stress is nothing new to most 40-year-old men. Chances are that in this "age of anxiety" (as W.H. Auden called it) such common "stressors" as job pressure, interpersonal relationships, bodily injury, pollution, noise, and other basic life situations have already tested a man's ability to react, thrive, and prosper. But for the man entering or already in his middle years, coping can sometimes become a more formidable task. Not only do the emotional stresses become more complex, but the years of physical wear and tear begin to be felt more acutely.

Dr. Hans Selye, the world's leading authority on stress, says that *"stress is the nonspecific response of the body to any demand made upon it,"* a definition kept deliberately loose so that it can encompass the fact that stress means different things to different people. For example, the prospect of performing in public might instill debilitating "stage fright" in one person while prompting another to summon up previously untapped resources of courage. This illustrates a point other researchers have made: **It is not events, but how people react to them, that causes stress.** The person who copes successfully with an intense demand—pleasant or unpleasant—reaps the psychological benefits (in the form of confidence and achievement) of having done so, while the person who does not cope as well experiences failure and depression (which may feed upon each other, further inhibiting the person's actions) as well as such physical discomforts as weakness, tension, and fatigue.

Most people know by now that stress is not something to be avoided. You can exert a great deal of control over your body's reaction to "stressors," lessening their ability to interfere with your well-being.

Though a wide variety of events and situations are considered stressful, studies have found that the body reacts in roughly the same way to each one. Adrenaline is released into the bloodstream, which hyperstimulates most of the body's sensory receptors. The stomach secretes hydrochloric acid, which —in the absence of food upon which to work—can burn tissue. Muscles become tense. If there is time for a person to evaluate and defuse a situation, the body will not go through these motions; however, such an evaluation might also lead to the "alarm reaction" if some form of danger is perceived. This state of heightened awareness is the body's way of preparing to fight.

The next stage is the crucial "fight or flight" response, in which a person either copes successfully with the stressful situation—in which cases the physical sensations are brought under control—or fails to cope. Over time, this failure leaves the body vulnerable to the numerous afflictions with which stress has been linked: cardiovascular disease, digestive problems (including ulcers), migraine headaches, and some say diminished resistance to infectious illnesses, and even cancer. **It is thus the goal of all stress control to develop effective coping behavior.**

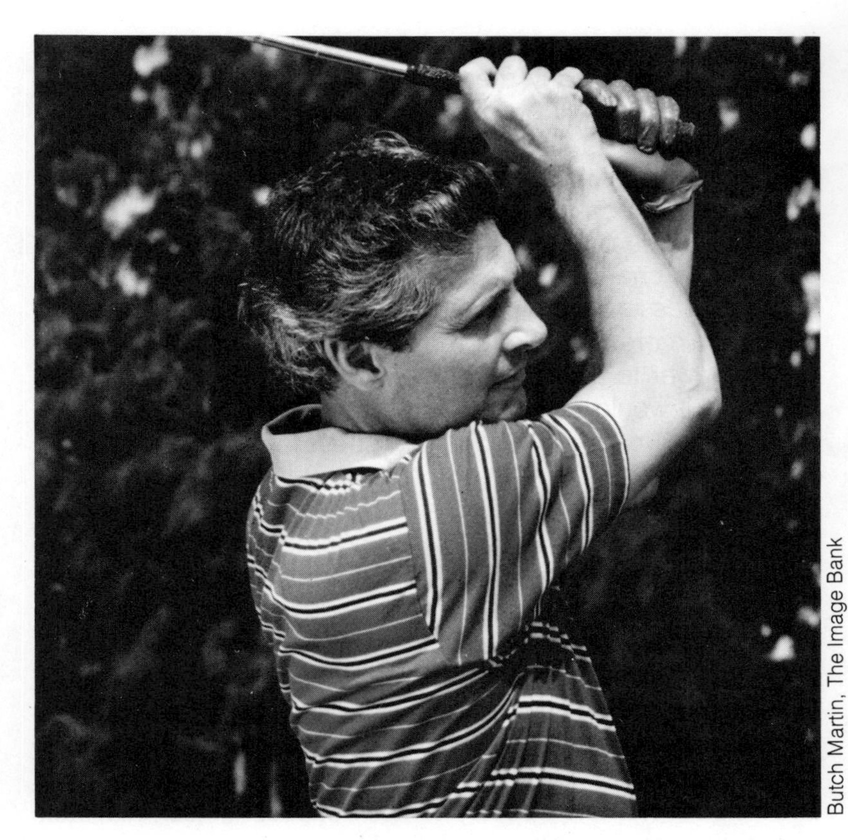

Butch Martin, The Image Bank

Both relaxation and exercise are a good way of combatting stress; for many men golf is the answer (and it burns 300 calories per hour).

The Mid-Life Crisis

Gail Sheehy, in her best-selling *Passages: Predictable Crises in Adult Life,* called it an "authenticity crisis." Others have called it the "plateau phenomenon" and the "mid-life crisis." Whatever the terminology, many men over 40 go through a period of reckoning in which they take stock of their achievements thus far in life and attempt to put themselves on a course for the future. But sometimes the future seems suddenly unclear. Undoubtedly, coping with this mental change is just as demanding as dealing with the physical exigencies of the body's age-related changes. This self-assessment can encompass a man's professional life, financial security, personal relations, and much more. Complex issues are involved that have considerable power to disrupt a man's life just when he might have imagined it would be coming together.

Being able to recognize potential stress factors is crucially important to waging effective control over stress and "mid-life crisis." The psychological factors should not be too difficult to identify, since they involve such fundamental aspects of life. Most likely, though, they will be accompanied by a host of physical disturbances—irritability, panic, fatigue, headaches, insomnia, intestinal distress, and general depression.

Even in the absence of any significant emotional quandaries—many men do sail through mid-life with nary a hint of crisis—these symptoms may indicate stress of a lesser (but still significant) magnitude: the feeling of intense pressures when facing deadlines at work, temporary sexual frustration, insomnia, lack of exercise, poor nutrition, and the like.

Doctors have also identified the "Type-A" personality, the hard-driving, competitive man seemingly always pressed for time, as something of a stress archetype. Such a man is considered two or three times more likely to suffer from a heart attack or to develop some other coronary condition. Obviously, this signifies an extreme lack of stress coping behavior. In fact, the Type-A man often relies on alcohol or tranquilizers to relieve stress, though of course no relief is really attained, as these "cures" only temporarily relieve the symptoms, not the causes, and at the same time accelerate the body's deterioration.

Stress Control

Stress control entails proper nutrition: Following a well-balanced diet (see Chapter Two) helps you avoid a nutritional deficiency which would make you more susceptible to illness, which obviously places a stress on the body. Then there are the widely marketed "stress vitamins," which usually contain vitamin C and vitamins of the B group. (You don't need these supplements if you're keeping to a proper diet.) You should also avoid caffeine, which in large amounts can increase your heart rate and anxiety. *Note:* While under any sort of job or personal pressure, try to refrain from dieting, which robs the body of energy and nutrients when it needs them most.

Stress control also includes proper exercise, which alleviates anxiety and helps relieve tension. Getting enough sleep, rest, and relaxation are, of course, the complements to exercise. Relaxation can take many forms. Lounging about the house or apartment is the simplest. (It's a good idea to take at least a few minutes every day to be idle.) The deep-breathing techniques of yoga have a tranquilizing effect on the body; and massage is good for relaxing strains in the body's musculature (a warm bath will do the same thing in a perhaps more indulgent fashion). Meditation is particularly good for clearing the mind of "clutter."

Biofeedback uses electronic sensors to teach a person to recognize and control the body's response to stress. Deep breathing, "positive visualization" (concentrating on pleasant thoughts, places, or sensations, and even listening to soothing music) are the methods then employed to actually bring about a relief from stress. (*Note:* You can utilize positive visualization and soothing music without doing biofeedback.) The relaxation response, a trained breathing technique, borrows from all of the above to achieve the same results. Among the more offbeat ways to fight stress is to spend about an hour in a "sensory deprivation chamber" or "deep tank"—a dark, almost womblike environment in which you soak for about an hour in a ten-inch-

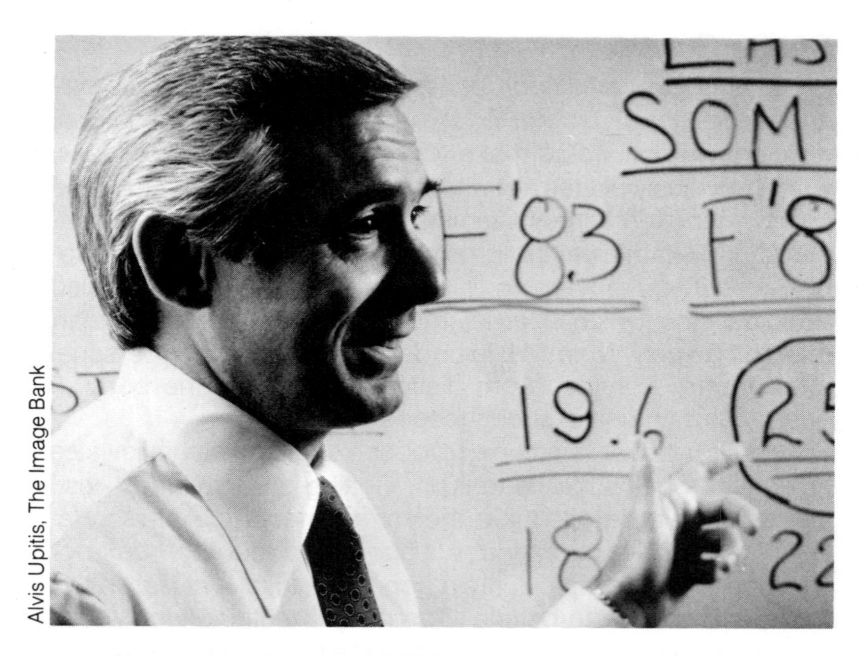

Alvis Upitis, The Image Bank

You can exercise your brain just as you do your body; sustained mental activity is one of the best ways to keep your brain working at any age.

deep solution of salt water, all the while oblivious of the hectic world outside.

Stress control often requires professional advice and attention—chances are there is a special stress-control organization in your area, or even a clinic at a local hospital. These can help you directly or guide you to the appropriate source of care.

Remember when under stress that it helps to talk your problems over with family and friends. If they can't help, consider seeing a professional. Whatever you do, don't rely on drugs—whether tranquilizers, sedatives, or alcohol—to cure anxiety and stress.

Finally, it is important to understand that stress is with us every day. If, as stress expert Selye has written, "the complete freedom from stress is death," then it is possible that the complete mastery of stress means life!

Brain Power

"You can't teach an old dog new tricks" is a familiar adage. Trouble is, that old saw just isn't true. Men over 40 do sometimes experience small memory lapses and other occasional difficulties that they might attribute to aging, but actually most of these cases of intellectual impairment are caused by general health and lifestyle factors (not by advancing age). There are age-related changes that occur in the brain, but these are not significant enough to seriously hamper a man's cognitive ability. One need only look at the late-in-life creative outpouring of Pablo Picasso, Albert Einstein, and George Bernard Shaw to see so-called "brain decline" for what it is: a myth. **Senility is not a sign of old age but a symptom of disease—dementia.**

As a man ages he loses billions of brain neurons, a staggering amount at first glance but actually just a small percentage of the total. There is also a decline in the number of dendritic spins—tiny filaments that help transmit information through the brain—but here, too, the loss is considered negligible. The speed with which nerve impulses are conducted falls by about

15 percent between the ages of 30 and 85—55 years is a long time—another gradual change thought to have relatively minor import. And finally, the brain as a whole gets slightly smaller over time; but this, too, has little effect on intellectual ability. Since these are the primary physical changes the aging brain undergoes, it can readily be seen that aging, in and of itself, does not impair brain function.

Recent scientific studies bear this out. One showed that 70-year-old men given problem-solving and concept-formation tests performed just as well as much younger individuals, provided they were given as much time as they needed to complete the tests; researchers stressed that although time pressure decreased performance levels—indicative of an age-linked "slowed response"—this should be distinguished from actual intellectual ability. An even more recent study showed that this problem could be overcome.

Meanwhile, a study focusing on memory loss found that this bugaboo could be traced not to the actual loss of any information but rather to an inability to retrieve it as well—a difficulty researchers thought might have to do with the sheer accumulation of data over time. The use of mnemonic devices produced a marked improvement in memory skills. These and other studies indicate that all the aging mind may need in order to perform up to its potential is practice.

True *dementia* strikes approximately 4 percent of the post-65 population. Roughly 50 percent is in the form of Alzheimer's disease, for which there is no cure nor known preventive treatment. Many other forms of dementia—including the form caused by a series of small strokes—can be prevented. How, then, can one take steps to preserve and prolong the mental edge?

Many factors contribute to the brain's health and welfare. The brain requires as much as thirty times more blood than other organs in order to function properly. It should be no surprise, then, that a good deal of age-related brain trouble is directly linked to the state of the body's blood vessels. The arteriosclerosis and hypertension that are so frequent at this age disrupt the blood and oxygen supply to the brain, resulting in a concomitant loss of thinking and reasoning skills.

One extensive study tracked its subjects for ten years and found that those men suffering from hypertension experienced a marked decline in intellectual performance. Aerobic exercise, which acts against the various cardiovascular diseases, helps supply oxygen and nutrients to the brain. And, not only does it have the added benefit of lessening tension and anxiety, which produce brain-weakening "mind clutter," but it also appears to improve short-term memory! A related causative factor—and one that is easily corrected—is that of poor posture; for instance, if you don't keep your neck and spine erect while sitting and working, choosing (probably unintentionally) instead to hang your head over your work or reading, the arteries feeding the brain are squeezed and your ability to think straight is restricted.

Proper nutrition is another primary factor in keeping the brain performing well. In addition to following a well-balanced diet, the B vitamins have been shown to influence memory and the ability to concentrate. For example, thiamine (vitamin B_1), found in pork, liver, pasta, cereals, bread, lima beans, and wheat germ, plays a role in the production of acetylcholine, a chemical that facilitates the transmission of nerve impulses through the brain. Iron, found in liver, carrots, fruit, whole wheat, and green vegetables, influences the workings of the brain's chemicals and pathways because of its role in assisting the transport of oxygen through the blood. Some of these brain foods (eggs, liver, and fish) also include choline, the substance from which vital acetylcholine is formed, and lecithin, which has been shown to maintain the health of membranes essential to message-relay functions. Following the same diet as that required for a healthy heart and arteries (see Chapter Two) is also recommended, since the most serious brain disorders—strokes—have most, if not all, of the same causative factors.

Finally, stimulation and challenge—hobbies, new pursuits,

and other forms of "mental exercise"—are crucial to keeping the brain active and will also help you live longer. By keeping both mentally and physically active and interacting with other people, you have your best chance of preserving your mental ability.

Strokes

The incidence of stroke—which has been called a "heart attack in the brain"—peaks at age 60, though it is not unknown for men in their 40s and 50s to have one. The Framingham Heart Study reports that more than 500,000 people suffer strokes each year, of which more than 156,000 (according to the AHA) died in 1983, making it the third leading cause of death after heart attack and cancer.

A stroke is actually a cardiovascular disease that disrupts or cuts off the flow of oxygen and nutrients to the brain. When the brain is denied these essentials, brain cells either die or cease to function, thus impairing the function—speech, memory, movement—that they control. A *cerebral thrombosis* occurs when there is an obstruction or clot in an artery supplying the brain. A *cerebral embolism* occurs if a loose clot in the bloodstream becomes lodged in an artery leading to the brain. The third main type of stroke, a *cerebral hemorrhage,* occurs when an artery in the brain ruptures, allowing blood to escape into the brain itself.

The AHA advises you to see your doctor if you experience any of the following warning signals for stroke, even in mild form. These symptoms may mean a major stroke is just days, weeks, or months away, or even that you've already experienced a "little stroke" (*transient ischemic attack,* also known as TIA), itself a precursor of a major attack.

- sudden, temporary weakness or numbness of the face, arm, and leg on one side of the body
- temporary loss of speech, or trouble speaking or understanding speech

- temporarily dimmed vision, or loss of vision, particularly in one eye
- unexplained dizziness, unsteadiness or sudden falls

Doctors will use an electroencephalogram (EEG), a spinal tap, an arteriogram, or a CAT scan (computerized axial tomographic scanner) to analyze warning signals and to examine people who have already suffered strokes. A general physical examination will also reveal such conditions as high blood pressure or other signs of heart disease, which is the major contributor to the occurrence of stroke.

Immediate treatment for stroke involves surgery, drugs, and hospital care. The prospects of rehabilitation depend mostly on the extent of the damage. Keep in mind, though, that severe harm to such basic skills as speech, memory, and movement is not easily repaired or restored, so most stroke victims should expect to suffer from persistent troubles.

The good news is that much can be done to prevent strokes from occurring in the first place. Since the conditions that cause stroke are similar if not identical to those that cause cardiovascular disease, a similar preventive program is in order (see Chapters One and Two). Smoking is also said to be a prominent factor. One Finnish study rated smokers fifteen times more likely to have strokes—the theory being that smoking reduces the elasticity of the blood vessels, eventually restricting the flow of blood to the brain. Finally, vigilance regarding the warning signals and the occurrence of TIA's is highly recommended.

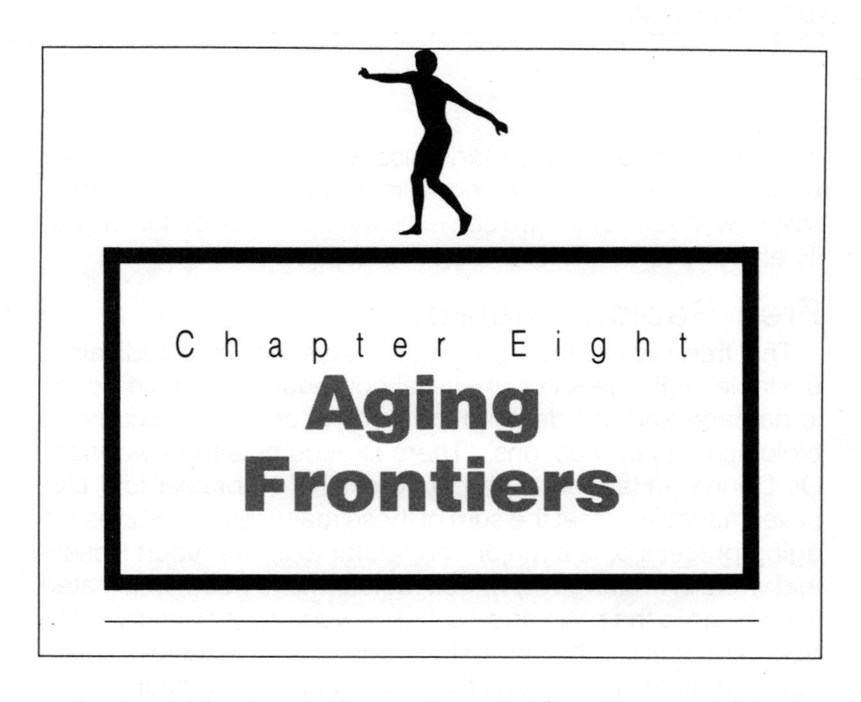

Chapter Eight
Aging Frontiers

"It should be the function of medicine to have people die young as late as possible" writes Ernst Wynder, epidemiologist and president of the American Health Foundation.

Most of this fitness guide has been devoted to exploring ways to prevent or adapt to the effects of aging, with the overriding goal being a vigorous, stimulating, physically uninhibited post-40 life. The American Association for the Advancement of Science recently predicted that the average life expectancy in the next century would reach 95 years, a significant increase but still short of what gerontologists think possible. When they predict that human beings will routinely live to 120 years of age and more, and that in the future a 90-year-old man will be the physical equivalent of today's 50-year-old, they are dead serious. These are not modern-day mad scientists, nor are they authors like Jules Verne and H.G. Welles fashioning stories based on wild hopes and private dreams of eternal youth, nor are they even Ponce de Leon types, searching for some magical fountain of youth. They are pioneers in the best sense of the word, who in fact have already made discoveries from which we can benefit. To speak of these people in a fitness book is to emphasize how much control we can exert over our chance for longevity and to offer a further impetus to action.

Free-Radical Therapy

The free-radical theory of aging says that free radicals—unstable, highly reactive chemical compounds—cause genetic damage and cell death in the body in constantly occurring biological chain reactions. "There is accumulating evidence," Dr. Denham Harman of the University of Nebraska told *Discover* magazine, "that the sum of these reactions constitutes the aging process or is a major contributor to it." As Albert Rosenfeld wrote in *Prolongevity II,* free radicals have been "implicated in damage to the brain and central nervous system, injury to the heart and cardiovascular system, and in the causation of cancer"—in other words, in all the leading causes of death.

Antioxidants are chemicals that apparently have the power to defuse the effects of free radicals by making them more chemically stable, and have thus become very popular as anti-aging agents. Vitamin E is an antioxidant, as are carotene, the mineral selenium (which can be toxic if taken in excess), and the food additive BHT (bis-hydroxytoluene).

Not all scientists are convinced of the validity of the free-radical theory, but it is nonetheless the leading example of a "wear and tear" theory of aging. These tend to see the body and its cells as being under continual attack over the course of a lifetime, finally succumbing when, as two other variations have it, the overall effect of a lifetime of "errors" becomes too much to bear, or when a few key genes—for instance, one that controls the cell's mechanism for repairing its DNA—fail to function as they should.

Clock Theories

The free-radical theory complements the "clock" theories of

aging. These say that the body is somehow preprogrammed to go through the aging cycle, to "self-destruct," so to speak, just as it was programmed to go through infancy, childhood, adolescence, and the earlier period of adulthood. Whether the clock "resides" in the brain (and is operated by the hypothalamus or the pituitary and thymus glands), works from within each cell, or functions through some combination of both is one of the major questions now under review.

One of the clock theories is actually a hormone clock theory and focuses on a so-called "death" or "killer" hormone secreted by the pituitary gland and known as DECO (for decreasing oxygen consumption hormone). It was discovered by W. Donner Denckla, whose studies showed that rats injected with the hormone showed signs of aging, while those whose pituitary was removed and who were then given other hormones showed delayed signs of aging. Following this lead, other researchers concentrated on another hormone, thymosine, which is secreted by the thyroid and which plays a part in helping the body's immune system stay strong. Since the thyroid begins to age as the rest of the body does, the thyroid-controlled immune system—and its eventual failure—is now seen as possibly comprising another of the body's "clocks" and thymosine as a possible antidote to degeneration.

Rather than choosing from among the many theories of aging, scientists are now suggesting that a combination of them is responsible for aging in what some call a "cascade" effect of interlinked causes and effects. In this scenario, the "clock" mechanism would be paramount, with the free radicals acknowledged as the primary cause of wear and tear.

What it boils down to is that while the scientists stay busy trying to understand the various aging clocks, **we the laymen should stay busy coping with the wear and tear.** We are powerful, resilient beings, with much more potential than we might realize. In fact, it is said that the brain's neurons could last as long as 150 to 200 years if only their support system—the body

—didn't give out so much sooner. We also have modern medicine—new treatments and new methods of early detection of disease, prosthetic devices and organ transplants, genetic engineering—doing its part in keeping human beings alive.

Another factor that might be most crucial for longevity is that our psychological selves catch up with our demonstrable physical prowess. As UCLA's Walford wrote, "Most people want to live long enough to grow old but at the same time dread old age!" Clearly, stimulation, a continued involvement in matters of purpose and meaning, and a belief in the heights that can be attained past the age of 40 are all crucial components of longevity. As long as the scientists' research remains just that—research—our minds and bodies are the best antidotes to aging we have.

Afterword

Your 40 Plus Life Begins Today!

We have seen what happens to a man's body as he grows older. We have also seen how most of these changes can be brought under control. We have even seen how the "life extenders" aim to redefine completely what it means to be over 40.

The body is our most precious possession, a source of myriad sensation and pleasure. As such, care should be lavished upon it; it should be worshipped or, better yet, simply taken care of and treated well.

Exercise. Proper nutrition. Attention paid to the rigors of life and how to lessen their effects. Give the body the respect due it, and in return it will bless its owner with the joys of life itself. What better incentive than this for the post-40 man to begin his new life today!